# MENTAL HEALTH AND PSYCHIATRIC NURSING

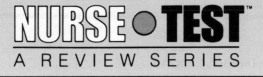

A REVIEW SERIES

# MENTAL HEALTH AND PSYCHIATRIC NURSING

**Linda E. Reese,** RN, MA
Deputy Chairperson and Assistant Professor of Nursing
College of Staten Island
Staten Island, N.Y.

**Series Editor**
**Laura Gasparis Vonfrolio,** RN, MA, CCRN, CEN
Assistant Professor of Nursing
College of Staten Island
Staten Island, N.Y.

Springhouse Corporation
Springhouse, Pennsylvania

# Staff

**Executive Director, Editorial**
Stanley Loeb

**Director of Trade and Textbooks**
Minnie B. Rose, RN, BSN, MEd

**Art Director**
John Hubbard

**Clinical Consultant**
Maryann Foley, RN, BSN

**Editors**
Diane Labus, Karen L. Zimmermann

**Copy Editors**
Mary Hohenhaus Hardy, Kate Daly

**Designers**
Stephanie Peters (associate art director), Julie Carleton Barlow,
Don Knauss

**Cover Illustration**
Marianne Hughes

**Manufacturing**
Deborah Meiris (manager), Anna Brindisi, T.A. Landis, Jennifer Suter

Printed in the United States of America.
NTQA4-011291

**Library of Congress Cataloging-in-Publication Data**
Reese, Linda E.
  Mental Health and psychiatric nursing / Linda E. Reese. p. cm. — (NurseTest)
  Includes bibliographical references and index.
  1. Psychiatric nursing—Examinations, questions, etc. I. Title. II. Series.
  [DNLM: 1. Psychiatric Nursing—examination questions. WY 18 R3295m]
RC440.R38 1991
610.73'68'076—dc20
DNLM/DLC                                      91-5211
0-87434-306-2                                      CIP

# Contents

# Consultant and Contributors

*Consultant*

**Jean Haspeslagh,** RN, DNS, Assistant Professor of Nursing, University of Southern Mississippi, Hattiesburg

*Contributors*

**Donna Kitun Allies,** RN, MN, PHN, CNP, Coordinator, Senior Medication Education Program, Santa Clara Health Department, Sunnyvale, Calif.

**Helene S. (Kay) Charron,** RN, MSN, Chairperson and Professor of Nursing, Monroe Community College, Rochester, N.Y.

**Madonna C. Coombs,** RN, MSN, MACE, Assistant Professor of Nursing, Marshall University, Huntington, W.V.

**Carol E. Garel,** RN, Adjunct Lecturer, College of Staten Island, N.Y.

**Carol Stier Goetz,** RN, MSN, CS, Instructor of Nursing, College of Staten Island, N.Y.

**Alice Geraghty Graham,** RN, BSN, MS, MA, Assistant Professor, College of Staten Island, N.Y.

**Janet S. Hickman,** RN, EdD, Associate Dean for Health Professions, Eastern College, St. Davids, Pa.

**Luzenia Howell Marques,** RN, EdD, Associate Professor of Nursing, Mobile (Ala.) College

**Kathleen Ryan Pappas,** RN, MA, CCS, CEAP, Instructor of Nursing, College of Staten Island, N.Y.

**Laurie Schretzlmeir,** RN, Nurse Specialist in Psychiatry, Private Practice, Manalapan, N.J.

**Nancy C. Seddio,** RN, PhD, CS, Psychotherapist, Private Practice, Staten Island, N.Y.

**Connie Spentz,** RN, MSN, Assistant Professor of Nursing, Erie Community College—City Campus, Buffalo, N.Y.

**Laura Gasparis Vonfrolio,** RN, MA, CCRN, CEN, Assistant Professor of Nursing, College of Staten Island, N.Y.

# Acknowledgments and Dedication

I begin by acknowledging Laura Gasparis Vonfrolio for her creativity, motivating energy, talent, and tremendous dedication to nursing that enabled me to complete this project. She is truly a gift to all of us.

I wish to thank my contributing authors for sharing their expertise to help make this book possible. Thanks also to my colleagues in the Department of Nursing at the College of Staten Island, who were so supportive and encouraging during this project.

A special thanks to Ethel Yauch, who showed tremendous patience and good humor in typing the manuscript. Her ability to translate my writing, endless arrows, and cut-and-pasted pages was truly appreciated.

---

To Tom for always believing in me;
Colin, my special creation;
and Ellen for always being there for me.

---

# Preface

This book is one in a series designed to help nursing students, professional licensed or registered nurses, nurses educated abroad, and nurses returning to the field improve their test-taking skills and increase their theoretical knowledge of nursing. It features case-study situations and a multiple-choice question-and-answer format similar to that used in NCLEX-RN (National Council Licensure Examination for Registered Nurses) and nursing challenge examinations. It also includes a comprehensive examination to test overall knowledge of questions and answers presented in each of the chapters.

*Mental Health and Psychiatric Nursing* offers theoretical and clinical information on the various topics covered in most mental health and psychiatric nursing textbooks and focuses on:
• understanding concepts essential to psychiatric nursing
• identifying the nurse's role in various treatment settings
• providing psychiatric care to those who are anxious or dangerous to self and others
• caring for patients with disruptions in relatedness or disordered mood
• providing psychosocial care for chronically ill patients and their families
• helping children, adolescents, and elderly patients with special psychosocial needs.

When using this book, remember to begin with the first question in each chapter and proceed in a sequential manner. Do not skip around; subsequent answers frequently build on previous ones.

# Introduction

Nurses are tested continually throughout their careers—as nursing students in the classroom, as professionals undergoing licensure or certification, and as practicing clinicians in the health care delivery field. Such testing helps to measure acquired knowledge and ultimately prepares nurses for real-life clinical situations.

Because testing knowledge is an important, ongoing aspect of a nurse's career and heavy emphasis is placed upon passing certain critical examinations, such as NCLEX-RN (National Council Licensure Examination for Registered Nurses) and nursing challenge examinations, nurses must rely on practical study guides and effective test-taking strategies if they are to succeed.

NurseTest: A Review Series was developed to help nurses improve their test-taking abilities and increase their general clinical knowledge. Each book in the series focuses on a specific area of study or a speciality of nursing practice. Written in a question-and-answer format, each book includes hundreds of questions built on case-study situations and a final comprehensive examination that tests overall subject knowledge. All questions, which appear at the beginning of each chapter, include four possible answers. The correct answers—along with rationales explaining why the correct answers are appropriate choices and why the incorrect answers are inappropriate—appear at the end of each chapter. A blank answer sheet is provided in each chapter.

Although having a thorough understanding of the clinical material is probably the best way to ensure a good test result, developing and implementing good test-taking strategies may mean the difference between passing and failing. Such strategies include physical and mental preparation, paying attention to directions, keeping track of the time, and reading the questions and answer choices carefully to determine the most appropriate response.

## Preparing for the test
Regardless of your reason for taking the test, you'll need to be prepared. If you are like many nurses, this may mean extensive reading, note taking, studying, and reviewing. Therefore, developing good study habits is key. Whether studying alone or in a group, you'll do well to follow a few simple rules:
- Find a place that is conducive to studying, such as a library, study hall, or lounge, if distractions are a problem.
- Limit your studying to several short sessions rather than one long cramming session.
- Highlight only the most essential information, and take selective notes.
- Concentrate on the most difficult or least familiar information first, saving the most familiar information for last.
- Anticipate feeling some anxiety over the test, but try to find ways to relieve it. For example, try practicing deep-breathing exercises and other forms of relaxation, such as rhythmically tensing and relaxing

muscle groups throughout your body. Practicing such exercises the night before the test and even while the papers are being distributed alleviates tension and promotes better concentration.

After what seems like countless hours of studying for an important test, the most effective final preparation is to relax and take it easy. Last-minute cramming can do little to increase knowledge and may cause unneeded stress and fatigue. Exercising or going to a movie the night before the test—then getting a good night's sleep—is usually most helpful.

**Taking the test**

Before answering any questions, remember to focus on the cardinal rules of test taking:

- Pay attention to directions.
- Read all instructions and questions carefully.
- Answer only what is being asked; do not read into a question anything beyond what is there.
- Know how much time is allotted for the test, and pace yourself accordingly. Be sure to note the halfway time.
- Scan the first page for a question you can answer easily, and mark the answer in the appropriate space on the answer sheet. Then go back to the first question and begin answering the questions in consecutive order. Answering an easy question first may give you a boost of confidence.
- Do not spend excessive time on any one question. If a question seems too difficult or complex, skip the question but remember to circle the number on the answer sheet; then return to the question after completing the other questions.
- Never leave an answer blank or mark two choices for the same answer.
- Compare the test to the answer sheet periodically to ensure that you haven't made any slight but costly errors, such as answering question 4 in question 5's space on the answer sheet.
- Erase all stray marks from the answer sheet before handing in the test.

**Choosing the correct response**

In a multiple-choice test, determining the correct answer to a question can sometimes be difficult. However, in many cases, you can successfully determine the correct answer by using one or more of the strategies listed below:

- Eliminate any obviously incorrect choices; then, reevaluate the remaining options and choose the most likely response. Ideally, you should try to narrow your choices to two likely option, affording yourself a 50% chance of choosing the correct answer. If choosing between the two remaining options seems especially difficult, take an educated guess.
- Look for key words or phrases in the question that can point to a correct response. For example, questions including the words "best," "most appropriate," or "most accurate" usually suggest that the correct response is a true statement, whereas those including "all...except," "least effective," and "least appropriate" usually suggest a false statement as the correct response. Such key words as "immediately,"

"promptly," and "highest priority" usually indicate that the correct response is something a nurse would normally do first.

- Look for interlocking clues, in which the correct response to one question forms the basis of the next question:

---

**1** The nurse is caring for Mr. P., who is exhibiting abnormal extension and adduction of the arms, pronation of the wrists, and flexion of the fingers. Which type of posturing is characterized by such abnormalities?

A. Decorticate
B. Apraxic
C. Akinetic
D. Decerebrate

---

**2** The nurse explains to Mr. P.'s daughter that decerebrate posturing typically results from:

A. Temporary lack of oxygen to the brain
B. Infection
C. Brain stem damage
D. Extrapyramidal system damage

---

In this example, "decerebrate" (the focus of the second question) is the correct answer to the first question. Although the mere repetition of "decerebrate" might suggest that it is the correct response, the real interlocking clue lies in the logical transition from one question to the other: in this case, the nurse cares for a patient exhibiting abnormal posturing, then explains the nature of such posturing to the patient's daughter.

*Important:* When looking for interlocking clues, always remember to read the questions and answer choices carefully, since choosing an answer solely on the basis of its repetition in another question can sometimes backfire:

---

**1** Which type of posturing is characterized by abnormal flexion and adduction of the arms and by flexion of the fingers and wrists on the chest?

A. Decorticate
B. Apraxic
C. Akinetic
D. Decerebrate

**2** The nurse understands that decerebrate posturing typically results from:
- **A.** Temporary lack of oxygen to the brain
- **B.** Infection
- **C.** Brain stem damage
- **D.** Extrapyramidal system damage

In this second example, "decerebrate" appears as an answer choice in the first question as well as the focus of the second question. Despite its repetition, however, "decerebrate" is not the correct response to the first question ("decorticate" is correct). The two questions are independent of each other, and no logical transition (or interlocking clue) exists.

**After the test**
Once you have completed the test, try to put it out of your mind; nothing can change the outcome at this point. Later, however, take time to review the test, if you're given an opportunity to do so—reviewing the questions and answers may provide some insight for future experiences. Otherwise, be satisfied with your accomplishment, and resume your usual work and leisure activities while you wait for the results. And expect to be pleasantly surprised.

**Alice Geraghty Graham,** RN, BSN, MS, MA
*Assistant Professor of Nursing*
*College of Staten Island*
*Staten Island, N.Y.*

# CHAPTER 1

# Foundations of Psychiatric Nursing

## Questions

**1** The nurse can use self-disclosure with a patient if:

A. She has experienced the same situation as the patient
B. The patient asks her directly about his experience
C. It helps the patient to talk more easily
D. It achieves a specific therapeutic goal

**2** The nurse who uses self-disclosure should:

A. Refocus on the patient's experience as quickly as possible
B. Allow the patient to ask questions about her experience
C. Discuss her experience in detail
D. Have the patient explain his perception of what the nurse has revealed

**3** During the mental status examination a patient may be asked to explain several proverbs, such as "Don't cry over spilled milk." The purpose is to evaluate the patient's ability to think:

A. Rationally
B. Concretely
C. Abstractly
D. Tangentially

**4** The terms *judgment* and *insight* sometimes are used incorrectly. Insight is the ability to:

A. Make appropriate choices
B. Control inappropriate impulses
C. Explain one's psychiatric diagnosis
D. Understand the nature of one's problem or situation

**5** The nurse documents, "The patient described her husband's abuse in an emotionless tone and with a flat facial expression." This statement describes the patient's:

A. Feelings
B. Blocking
C. Mood
D. Affect

**6** Although a patient changes topics quickly while relating his past psychiatric history, the nurse is able to follow his thoughts. The patient's pattern of thinking is called:

**A.** Looseness of association
**B.** Flight of ideas
**C.** Tangential thinking
**D.** Circumstantial thinking

**7** The nurse who suspects that a patient's behavior has a cultural basis should:

**A.** Read several articles about the patient's culture
**B.** Ask staff members of a similar culture about the patient's behavior
**C.** Observe the patient and his family and friends interacting with each other and other staff members
**D.** Accept the patient's behavior because it is probably culturally based

**8** Which contribution of the psychoanalytic model is particularly useful to psychiatric nurses?

**A.** All behavior has meaning
**B.** Behavior that is reinforced will be perpetuated
**C.** The first 6 years of a person's life determine his personality
**D.** Behavioral deviations result from an incongruence between verbal and nonverbal communication

**9** According to Freud's psychosexual theory, the ego has several functions, one of which is to:

**A.** Serve as the source of instinctual drives
**B.** Stimulate psychic energy
**C.** Operate as a conscience that controls unacceptable drives
**D.** Test reality and direct behavior

**10** Erikson described the psychosocial tasks of the developing person in his theoretical model. The primary developmental task of the young adult (age 18 to 25) is:

**A.** Intimacy versus isolation
**B.** Industry versus inferiority
**C.** Generativity versus stagnation
**D.** Trust versus mistrust

**11** Which of the following is a generally accepted criterion of mental health?

A. Self-acceptance
B. Absence of anxiety
C. Ability to control others
D. Happiness

**12** The basis for a therapeutic nurse-patient relationship begins with the nurse's:

A. Sincere desire to help others
B. Acceptance of others
C. Self-awareness and understanding
D. Sound knowledge of psychiatric nursing

**13** Which of the following should occur during the working phase of the nurse-patient relationship?

A. The nurse assesses the patient's needs and develops a plan of care for the patient
B. The nurse and the patient together evaluate and modify the goals of the relationship
C. The nurse and the patient discuss their feelings regarding the termination of the relationship
D. The nurse and the patient explore each other's expectations of the relationship

**14** The nurse should introduce information about the end of the nurse-patient relationship:

A. During the orientation phase
B. As the goals of the relationship are reached
C. At least one or two sessions before the last meeting
D. When the patient is able to tolerate it

**15** One example of the psychiatric nurse's role in primary prevention is:

A. Handling crisis intervention in an outpatient setting
B. Visiting the patient's home to discuss medication management
C. Conducting a postdischarge support group
D. Providing sex education classes for adolescents

**16** The most effective way for the nurse to set limits for a newly admitted patient who puts out his cigarettes on the dayroom floor is to:

**A.** Restrict the patient's smoking to times when he can be closely supervised by a staff member
**B.** Encourage other patients to speak with the patient about dirtying the dayroom floor
**C.** Ask the patient if he puts out his cigarettes on the floor at home
**D.** Hand the patient an ashtray and tell him he must use it or he will not be allowed to smoke

**17** A busy woman attorney with a successful law practice is admitted to the acute care hospital with epigastric pain. Since admission, she has called the nurse every 15 minutes with one request or another. The patient is exhibiting:

**A.** Repression
**B.** Somatization
**C.** Regression
**D.** Conversion

**18** G. lost an important advertising account and had a flat tire on the way home. That evening, he began to find fault with everyone. Which defense mechanism is he using?

**A.** Displacement
**B.** Projection
**C.** Regression
**D.** Sublimation

**19** Which primary unconscious defense mechanism keeps highly anxiety-producing situations out of conscious awareness?

**A.** Introjection
**B.** Regression
**C.** Repression
**D.** Denial

**20** J., age 17, rarely expresses his feelings and usually remains passive; however, when he is angry, his face typically becomes flushed and his blood pressure rises to 170/100 mm Hg. His parents are described as passive and easygoing. J. may be using which defense mechanism to handle his anger?

**A.** Displacement
**B.** Introjection
**C.** Projection
**D.** Sublimation

## SITUATION

*F., age 18, returns home from school to discover that her mother has been in a serious automobile accident.*

*Questions 21 to 23 refer to this situation.*

**21** F. initially responds to the news by yelling, "No, I don't believe it. It can't be true." F. is using which defense mechanism?

**A.** Introjection
**B.** Suppression
**C.** Denial
**D.** Repression

**22** F. excuses herself from the hospital to go home by saying to her father, "I have to go home. I can't stay awake anymore, and I've been here most of the day." Which defense mechanism is F. using?

**A.** Reaction formation
**B.** Rationalization
**C.** Denial
**D.** Regression

**23** On arriving home, F. encounters neighbors who ask about her mother's condition. F. tells them all the details unemotionally and without feeling upset. This behavior illustrates her use of:

**A.** Displacement
**B.** Introjection
**C.** Intellectualization
**D.** Conversion

## SITUATION

*W., a 27-year-old secretary, is brought to the hospital in an agitated state. She is admitted to the psychiatric unit for observation and treatment.*

*Questions 24 to 29 refer to this situation.*

**24** The nurse enters W.'s room for the first time and says, "W., I'm E., the nurse. I'll help you get settled." W. responds, "I want another nurse. I don't like you. You're mean." The nurse recognizes that W.'s response is an example of:

**A.** Identification
**B.** Regression
**C.** Countertransference
**D.** Transference

**25** Before responding to W.'s initial outburst, the nurse should:

**A.** Make sure she is a safe distance from the patient
**B.** Move closer to the patient to show that she is not afraid
**C.** Assess her own feelings and responses to the patient's behavior
**D.** Recognize that it takes time for relationships to develop and not feel hurt

**26** What would be the most therapeutic initial response by the nurse?

**A.** Say nothing, accept what the patient has said, and remain nearby
**B.** Say, "W., we've just met. Why do you think I'm mean?"
**C.** Say, "I'm only trying to be helpful. Let me help you put your things away"
**D.** Say, "I'll be back in half an hour," then leave the patient's room

**27** As W. puts her things away, she talks rapidly and folds and unfolds her clothes several times. She cannot seem to settle down. Which nursing diagnostic category is most applicable initially?

**A.** Self-care deficit
**B.** Anxiety
**C.** Impaired verbal communication
**D.** Powerlessness

**28** The nurse needs to complete W.'s admission interview. In light of the patient's initial behavior, which nursing approach is best?

**A.** Allow W. as much time as she needs to arrange her clothes and belongings
**B.** Recognize that W. is upset, but stress that the admission interview must be completed
**C.** Tell W. that her repetitious behavior is interfering with the interview and that she must stop and cooperate
**D.** Suggest that W. finish arranging her belongings later, and mention that she needs to complete her admission interview

**29** The best way to continue W.'s mental status interview is to ask:

**A.** "Why are you here, W.?"
**B.** "What events led to your coming to the hospital?"
**C.** "What do you want us to do for you while you are here?"
**D.** "Tell me about your family, W."

## SITUATION

*V., age 40, is admitted to the medical unit for treatment of a peptic ulcer.*

*Questions 30 and 31 refer to this situation.*

**30** A nursing assistant remarks, "I don't know what's wrong with V. He never looks at me when I talk to him. He just stares at the floor." How should the nurse respond to the nursing assistant?

**A.** "I wouldn't worry about it. That's just how some people are"
**B.** "When I give him his medication, I'll ask him if he is aware that he does this"
**C.** "You need to develop more patience with V. It takes time for patients to feel at ease in the hospital"
**D.** "What seems to bother you most about V.'s not looking at you?"

**31** The nurse can help the nursing assistant understand patient responses that are different from her own by explaining the importance of:

**A.** Accepting the patient's way of responding and treat all patients alike
**B.** Suppressing any feelings of discomfort or anxiety that the patient's behaviors create
**C.** Evaluating behaviors in the context of the patient's cultural background
**D.** Confronting the patient about his behaviors in order to understand their meaning

## SITUATION

*The nurse has been caring for G., a 58-year-old chronic paranoid schizophrenic patient, for several months. She has held several one-to-one sessions with him. During this particular session, he appears more anxious than usual.*

*Questions 32 to 36 refer to this situation.*

**32** At the beginning of the session, G. speaks quite rapidly and loudly. This behavior indicates a possible change in which form of nonverbal communication?

**A.** Appearance
**B.** Kinesics
**C.** Paralanguage
**D.** Proxemics

**33** Still speaking loudly, G. says, "Speak up! You talk too softly. Who could carry on a conversation with someone who sounds like a squeaky little mouse?" According to Berne's theory of communication, the patient is communicating from which "ego state"?

A. Parent
B. Adult
C. Adolescent
D. Child

**34** Besides his loud, rapid speech, G. swings his feet and rapidly taps his fingers on the arm of the chair. Yet he says, "I certainly feel calm today. I didn't know life could be so tranquil." Which response by the nurse is most appropriate?

A. "I'm glad to hear you are feeling calm and settled this morning"
B. "You tell me that you are calm, but your body seems to be sending a different message"
C. "I think we should talk about how calm the weather is today"
D. "I'm glad you are feeling so calm. Things will be better for you now—you can count on that"

**35** G.'s anxiety level takes a toll on the nurse, and she feels her body tensing. The nurse momentarily questions the therapeutic quality of her listening skills. Which behavior on the nurse's part indicates her decreased attention to G.'s problems?

A. Moving her chair so she directly faces G.
B. Leaning forward toward G.
C. Maintaining direct eye contact
D. Crossing her arms and legs

**36** Which statement is most appropriate to end the one-to-one session with G.?

A. "Your body seems more relaxed now, G."
B. "Today we talked about how your body can provide clues to your feelings"
C. "Did you think today's session was of value to you?"
D. "I'm going to lunch now; our time is up"

---

### SITUATION

*D., age 21, has just been admitted to the inpatient psychiatric unit. Her facial expression indicates severe panic, and she repeatedly states, "I know the police are going to shoot me. They found out that I'm the daughter of the devil."*

*Questions 37 to 39 refer to this situation.*

---

**37** To initiate a therapeutic nurse-patient relationship with D., the nurse should say:

**A.** "You certainly look stressed, D. Can you tell me about the up-setting events that have occurred in your life recently?"
**B.** "Hello, my name is A. I'm a nurse, and I will care for you when I am on duty. Would you like me to call you D., or do you prefer something else?"
**C.** "You are having very frightening thoughts. I will help you find ways to cope with this scary thinking"
**D.** "Hello, D. I am going to be caring for you while I am on duty. You look very frightened, but by tomorrow I,m sure you'll feel better"

---

**38** After the assessment and intake procedures are completed, the nurse explains that she will try to be available to talk with D. when needed and that she will spend time with her each morning from 10:00 until 10:30 in a specific corner of the dayroom. The main rationale for communicating these planned nursing interventions is to:

**A.** Provide a structured environment for D.
**B.** Instill hope in D.
**C.** Attempt to establish a trusting relationship
**D.** Provide time for completing nursing responsibilities

**39** During the first few one-to-one sessions, D. seems eager to talk, discusses her problems readily, and makes great efforts to focus on and describe her experiences. Then she begins to "forget" to come to scheduled sessions. When she does come, she seems suspicious and reluctant to talk. What is the most likely explanation for her behavior?

**A.** D. is fearful that she has revealed too much and that the nurse will now reject her; she is temporarily retreating to a safe distance
**B.** D. has found one-to-one sessions to be too personally intrusive and is attempting to protect her privacy
**C.** D.'s suspiciousness indicates that her symptoms have not responded to treatment and that her medication should be reevaluated
**D.** D. and the nurse are in a personality conflict, and the nurse should consider transferring the patient to another primary nurse

# Answer sheet

|   | A | B | C | D |   |   | A | B | C | D |
|---|---|---|---|---|---|---|---|---|---|---|
| 1 | ○ | ○ | ○ | ○ |   | 31 | ○ | ○ | ○ | ○ |
| 2 | ○ | ○ | ○ | ○ |   | 32 | ○ | ○ | ○ | ○ |
| 3 | ○ | ○ | ○ | ○ |   | 33 | ○ | ○ | ○ | ○ |
| 4 | ○ | ○ | ○ | ○ |   | 34 | ○ | ○ | ○ | ○ |
| 5 | ○ | ○ | ○ | ○ |   | 35 | ○ | ○ | ○ | ○ |
| 6 | ○ | ○ | ○ | ○ |   | 36 | ○ | ○ | ○ | ○ |
| 7 | ○ | ○ | ○ | ○ |   | 37 | ○ | ○ | ○ | ○ |
| 8 | ○ | ○ | ○ | ○ |   | 38 | ○ | ○ | ○ | ○ |
| 9 | ○ | ○ | ○ | ○ |   | 39 | ○ | ○ | ○ | ○ |
| 10 | ○ | ○ | ○ | ○ |   |   |   |   |   |   |
| 11 | ○ | ○ | ○ | ○ |   |   |   |   |   |   |
| 12 | ○ | ○ | ○ | ○ |   |   |   |   |   |   |
| 13 | ○ | ○ | ○ | ○ |   |   |   |   |   |   |
| 14 | ○ | ○ | ○ | ○ |   |   |   |   |   |   |
| 15 | ○ | ○ | ○ | ○ |   |   |   |   |   |   |
| 16 | ○ | ○ | ○ | ○ |   |   |   |   |   |   |
| 17 | ○ | ○ | ○ | ○ |   |   |   |   |   |   |
| 18 | ○ | ○ | ○ | ○ |   |   |   |   |   |   |
| 19 | ○ | ○ | ○ | ○ |   |   |   |   |   |   |
| 20 | ○ | ○ | ○ | ○ |   |   |   |   |   |   |
| 21 | ○ | ○ | ○ | ○ |   |   |   |   |   |   |
| 22 | ○ | ○ | ○ | ○ |   |   |   |   |   |   |
| 23 | ○ | ○ | ○ | ○ |   |   |   |   |   |   |
| 24 | ○ | ○ | ○ | ○ |   |   |   |   |   |   |
| 25 | ○ | ○ | ○ | ○ |   |   |   |   |   |   |
| 26 | ○ | ○ | ○ | ○ |   |   |   |   |   |   |
| 27 | ○ | ○ | ○ | ○ |   |   |   |   |   |   |
| 28 | ○ | ○ | ○ | ○ |   |   |   |   |   |   |
| 29 | ○ | ○ | ○ | ○ |   |   |   |   |   |   |
| 30 | ○ | ○ | ○ | ○ |   |   |   |   |   |   |

## Answers and rationales

**1** Correct answer—**D**

Self-disclosure, making personal statements about oneself, can be a useful tool for the nurse. However, the nurse should use self-disclosure judiciously and with a specific therapeutic purpose in mind. The nurse should listen to the patient closely and remember that experiences are sometimes similar but never the same for different people. Too many self-disclosures can shift the focus from the patient to the nurse. Self-disclosure that distracts the patient from treatment issues does not benefit the patient and may alienate him from the nurse.

**2** Correct answer—**A**

The nurse's self-disclosure should be brief and to the point so that the interaction can be refocused on the patient's experience. Because the patient is the focus of the nurse-patient relationship, the nurse should not dwell upon her experience.

**3** Correct answer—**C**

Abstract thinking is the ability to conceptualize and interpret meaning. It is a higher level of intellectual functioning than concrete thinking, in which the patient would explain the proverb by its literal meaning. Rational thinking involves the ability to think logically, make judgments, and be goal directed. Tangential thinking is scattered, non-goal-directed, and difficult to follow. Patients with such conditions as organic brain disease and schizophrenia typically are unable to conceptualize and comprehend abstract meaning. They interpret such statements as "Don't cry over spilled milk" in a literal sense, such as "Even if you spill your milk, you shouldn't cry about it."

**4** Correct answer—**D**

Insight is the degree to which the patient understands a situation or problem and its effect on his life. Judgment is the ability to make decisions and behave in an appropriate manner. Although a patient may be able to explain his psychiatric diagnosis, he may not have enough insight to understand the underlying problem and how it is affecting his life.

## 5 Correct answer—D

Affect refers to one's emotional expression, in this case the manner in which the patient talks about her experiences. Feelings are emotional states or perceptions. Blocking describes the interruption of thoughts. Moods are prolonged emotional states expressed by the affect.

## 6 Correct answer—B

Flight of ideas describes a thought pattern in which a patient moves rapidly from one topic to the next with some connection. Looseness of association describes a pattern in which no logical connection between ideas is apparent. Tangential thoughts seem to be related but miss the point. A circumstantial thought pattern is exhibited when a patient talks around the subject and includes much unnecessary information.

## 7 Correct answer—C

Assessing the patient's interactions with others helps to determine whether the behavior is part of his usual pattern. It also may help the nurse to understand the meaning of the behavior for this particular patient. Reading about a different culture, consulting other staff members, and talking with the patient also are helpful once the nurse has observed the patient's interaction with others. Although the nurse must be able to accept the patient as an individual, she need not accept behaviors that are unhealthy or inappropriate. The nurse should work with the patient to better understand the cultural differences and to help him change any unhealthy or unacceptable behaviors, such as unwarranted sexual advances.

## 8 Correct answer—A

The principle that all behavior has meaning is of particular importance to the psychiatric nurse. It is the basis for the nurse's assessment and analysis of the patient's behavior, which reflects his needs. Psychoanalytic theory also proposes that the first 6 years of a person's life determine his later personality. These early influences are difficult if not impossible to counteract. However, this assumption is less useful to the nurse in planning interventions that meet the patient's current needs. Reinforcement as a means of perpetuating behavior is associated with behavioral theory, not the psychoanalytic model. Similarly, incongruence between verbal and nonverbal communications is a part of communications theory.

**9** Correct answer—**D**

The ego tests reality and directs behavior by mediating between the pleasure-seeking instinctual drives of the id and the restrictiveness of the superego. The superego also is called the conscience. The id is the source of psychic energy.

**10** Correct answer—**A**

The primary developmental task of the young adult is to develop intimacy with another person while making choices about relationships and career. Industry, a task associated with 6- to 12-year-olds, involves active socialization as the child moves from family into society; much of the child's energy is focused on acquiring competency. Generativity is associated with middle age and is characterized by parental responsibility and concern for future generations. The task of trust is typical of infancy. It is accomplished when the infant receives adequate mothering and his oral needs are met.

**11** Correct answer—**A**

Self-acceptance is a generally accepted criterion of mental health and serves as the basis for healthy relationships with others. Some degree of anxiety is necessary to stimulate growth and adaptation. Self-control and self-direction rather than the ability to control others are indicative of mental health. Happiness, though desirable, is not an effective indicator of mental health because even mentally healthy people are unhappy when faced with such events as illness, loss, and death.

**12** Correct answer—**C**

Although all the choices are certainly desirable, knowledge of self serves as the basis for building a strong therapeutic nurse-patient relationship. The nurse must be aware of and understand her feelings and behavior before she can understand and help others.

**13** Correct answer—**B**

The therapeutic nurse-patient relationship consists of four phases: preinteraction, introduction or orientation, working, and termination. In the working phase, the nurse and the patient together evaluate and refine the goals established in the orientation phase. In addition, major therapeutic work takes place, and insight is integrated into a plan of action. The orientation phase involves assessing the patient, formulating a contract, exploring feelings, and establishing expectations about the relationship. In the termination phase, the nurse prepares the patient for separation and explores feelings about the end of the relationship.

## 14 Correct answer—A

Preparation for ending the nurse-patient relationship begins during the orientation phase, when the limits of the relationship are established. Termination also should be discussed as goals are achieved and the relationship nears an end. Although the nurse should remind the patient that only one or two sessions are left, she must not wait until then to prepare the patient for the relationship's termination. Waiting until the patient can tolerate ending the relationship also is too late. Because many patients have had negative experiences when ending relationships, the nurse can use termination of the nurse-patient relationship to prepare the patient for—and work him through—positive termination experiences with others.

## 15 Correct answer—D

The psychiatric nurse participates in primary, secondary, and tertiary prevention activities. Primary prevention includes providing sex education classes for adolescents and education programs that promote mental health and prevent future psychiatric episodes. Secondary prevention involves treatment to reduce psychiatric problems. Crisis intervention in an outpatient setting is one example of secondary prevention. Administering and supervising medication regimens and participating in the therapeutic milieu are other means of secondary prevention. Tertiary prevention involves helping patients who are recovering from psychiatric illness; activities that are directed toward providing aftercare and rehabilitation are part of this role. Conducting a postdischarge support group is a tertiary prevention activity.

## 16 Correct answer—D

Setting limits is necessary to help patients behave in socially acceptable ways. By handing the patient an ashtray and clearly stating that he must use it or he will not be allowed to smoke, the nurse is setting limits on his behavior. Because he is a newly admitted patient, the nurse may need to restate these limits in a manner that shows disapproval of the behavior but does not reject him as a person. A matter-of-fact, nonpunitive tone of voice is important. If the patient does not comply, he must face the consequences, in this case, not to be allowed to smoke. If the patient's mental status is such that he cannot understand or follow these limits, his smoking may need to be supervised. Encouraging other patients to deal with a new patient is not advisable. Asking the patient if he puts out cigarettes on the floor at home has no bearing on whether this behavior is acceptable in the hospital.

## 17 Correct answer—C

The patient is exhibiting the defense mechanism of regression—a return to behaviors characteristic of an earlier developmental level. Her dependent, attention-getting behavior is an attempt to relieve anxiety. Repression would be evidenced by ignoring the symptoms. Somatization is the channeling of anxiety into a preoccupation with physical complaints. Conversion involves the transfer of a mental conflict into a physical symptom to relieve anxiety.

## 18 Correct answer—A

G. is using displacement, a mechanism in which the patient discharges his feelings of anger and rejection in an indirect way that he perceives as safe—in this situation, by displacing his anger from work and car problems onto family members. Projection is attributing one's emotions to—or blaming them on—others. Regression is a retreat to earlier levels of developmental behavior to relieve anxiety. Sublimation is a socially acceptable discharge of psychic energy or anger, such as through exercise or some other productive activity.

## 19 Correct answer—C

Repression, the unconscious exclusion of painful or conflicting thoughts, impulses, or memories from awareness, is the primary ego defense. Other defense mechanisms tend to reinforce the anxiety. Introjection is an intense identification in which an individual incorporates another person's or group's values or qualities into his own ego structure. Regression is a retreat into an earlier developmental level in a time of stress. Denial is avoidance of unpleasant realities by ignoring them.

## 20 Correct answer—B

J. may be introjecting his parents' belief that anger should not be outwardly expressed. He also may be holding in his angry feelings, as evidenced by his increased blood pressure. (Increased blood pressure is a common physiologic reaction to the fight-or-flight response brought on by strong emotions. Habitual failure to express anger may contribute to hypertension.) Displacement is the discharge of negative feelings onto another person or an object. Projection is the attribution of one's own thoughts or impulses to another person. Sublimation is the channeling of unbearable or socially unacceptable behaviors to more socially acceptable outlets.

## 21 Correct answer—C

Denial is the avoidance of reality by ignoring or refusing to acknowledge unpleasant incidents. This defense mechanism is used to allay anxiety immediately following a stressful event. Introjection is an intense form of identification in which a person incorporates the values or qualities of another person or group into his own ego structure. Suppression is the conscious analog of repression. A person uses suppression intentionally and consciously excludes material from awareness. Repression is the unconscious exclusion of painful episodes from awareness.

## 22 Correct answer—B

Rationalization is the offering of a socially acceptable or logical reason for doing, feeling, or behaving in a way that might not be otherwise acceptable. Reaction formation is the development of attitudes or behaviors that are opposite of what one actually feels or wants to do. Denial is avoiding reality by ignoring unpleasant events. Regression is a return to behaviors that reflect an earlier developmental level.

## 23 Correct answer—C

Intellectualization is the splitting off of the emotional part of an idea, impulse, or act. The emotional aspect then is repressed, either temporarily or over the long term. Displacement is discharging feelings in an indirect way perceived as safe. Introjection is an intense identification in which an individual incorporates another person's or group's values or qualities into his own ego structure.

Conversion is the transfer of a mental conflict into a physical symptom.

## 24 Correct answer—D

When a patient's response to the nurse is extremely negative or extremely positive with no apparent basis, transference of feelings from another relationship is probably occurring. If the nurse has similar unwarranted responses to the patient, countertransference is taking place. Identification is a defense mechanism in which the patient adopts the characteristics of the nurse. Regression is a retreat to behaviors manifested during an earlier developmental level.

## 25 Correct answer—C

The nurse must first identify her feelings toward the patient and use them as a guide to determine an appropriate response. An accurate assessment of the distance needed between the nurse and the patient is possible only if the nurse assesses her own response first. The nurse's recognition that trust takes time to develop may be useful in planning an appropriate response; however, the nurse should identify her feelings about the patient before formulating a response.

## 26 Correct answer—A

Displaying an accepting attitude of the patient's negative response helps foster trust. It also demonstrates the nurse's interest in and concern for the patient without challenging the patient, denying the patient's feelings, or leaving the patient alone. The patient probably cannot verbalize why she feels the way she does; challenging her will only increase her anxiety and make her feel more vulnerable. By emphasizing that she is only being helpful, the nurse implies that the patient's feelings are erroneous. Leaving the room serves no purpose and may exacerbate the patient's anxiety by increasing her feelings of aloneness and introducing a feeling of desertion.

## 27 Correct answer—B

Anxiety is an appropriate nursing diagnostic category initially because the patient's behavior mimics some of the objective signs of anxiety, which include restlessness, irritability, rapid speech, inability to complete tasks, and verbal expressions of tension. The other diagnostic categories—Self-care deficit, Impaired verbal communication, and Powerlessness—are premature because the nurse has not had an opportunity to complete a thorough nursing assessment.

## 28 Correct answer—D

Establishing priorities and communicating them to the patient in a clear, nonjudgmental way is important. Suggesting that the patient can continue her activities later demonstrates acceptance of the patient's behavior yet helps the nurse complete the admission interview in a timely manner. Emphasizing the nurse's need to complete the interview shifts the focus from the patient to the nurse.

## 29 Correct answer—B

Obtaining the patient's perspective of the events leading to her admission is an excellent source of assessment data. "Why" questions should be avoided because they require analysis of the problem and often produce anxiety. Finding out about the patient's family and her goals for treatment are important but should be discussed later.

## 30 Correct answer—D

Effective communication is based on self-understanding. Exploring the nursing assistant's feelings and responses to the patient's behavior facilitates the development of self-awareness, a prerequisite to planning a therapeutic response. Denying the assistant's feelings of frustration without exploring their cause or intervening with the patient on behalf of the assistant at this point would not be helpful to the assistant. Asking the assistant to have more patience may stop her from exploring her feelings about the situation. By exploring the assistant's feelings, the nurse can help her understand the mental health needs of the patient.

## 31 Correct answer—C

To assess the patient's needs, the nursing assistant must take into account the patient's cultural influences, values, beliefs, attitudes, and verbal and nonverbal behavior. In some cultures, looking down is a sign of respect. All patients are different and should be treated as individuals. The nurse should encourage the assistant to discuss her discomfort or anxiety rather than supress it. She should not recommend confronting the patient because this will cause him to feel alientated.

## 32 Correct answer—C

Paralanguage is the use of vocal effects, such as tone and tempo, to convey a message. Appearance is to the way people look. Kinesics involves body language or movement. Proxemics is the use of spatial relationships (distance between people) during interaction to communicate meaning.

## 33 Correct answer—A

The Transactional Analysis Model consists of three ego states— parent, adult, and child. Each ego state is unique, yet all three combine to form one personality. Berne's parent ego state includes the aspects of critical parent and nurturing parent. G. sounds like a "critical parent" and therefore is communicating from the parent ego state. A patient communicating from the child ego state would exhibit feelings formulated during childhood, such as fear of authority figures. A patient communicating from the adult ego state would appear rational and capable of coping with feelings and situations in a logical manner. Berne's theory does not include an adolescent ego state.

## 34 Correct answer—B

Using confrontation to call attention to the discrepancy between what the patient says (verbal communication) and how he behaves (nonverbal communication) can help the patient become aware of his true feelings. Nonverbal behavior usually is a more precise indicator of feelings. Responses that ignore the incongruent behavior are not therapeutic.

## 35 Correct answer—D

Crossing the arms and legs can be a sign of defensiveness and decreased involvement with others. Signs of attentiveness and interest include facing another person squarely, leaning forward, and maintaining direct eye contact.

## 36 Correct answer—B

Summarizing at the end of a one-to-one session helps reinforce the most significant information discussed. Observations about how relaxed the patient appears are more appropriate during the session. Questions that elicit a "Yes" or "No" response are generally nontherapeutic to the patient. The nurse's telling the patient that she is now going to lunch does not focus on the patient and is therefore inappropriate.

## 37 Correct answer—**B**

The first task during the introductory, or orientation, phase of the nurse-patient relationship is to formulate a contract, which begins with the exchange of names and an explanation of the roles and limits of the relationship. These tasks should precede the exploration of relevant stressors and new coping mechanisms. Offering false reassurance is never therapeutic.

## 38 Correct answer—**C**

Availability, reliability, and consistency are critical factors in establishing trust with patients. Being specific about the time and place of meetings helps establish trust, which is the initial main objective. Although important, structuring the environment and instilling hope are not the primary tasks at this time. Arranging a regular meeting with the patient allows the nurse to plan her work load, but it is not a major reason for such scheduling.

## 39 Correct answer—**A**

Patients often are fearful that if they reveal themselves initially, the nurse will reject them, as others have done in the past. D. may or may not be aware that she is pulling back from the nurse. Her behavior actually is an indication of her potential to trust and should be considered a normal response at this point in the nurse-patient relationship. No evidence exists to support the other explanations.

# CHAPTER 2

# The Nurse's Role in Psychiatric Settings

# Questions

*A., age 15, is admitted to the unit for chronic psychiatric patients. This unit uses a token economy system as its treatment modality.*

*Questions 1 to 4 refer to this situation.*

**1** A token economy system is based on the principles of:

**A.** Psychoanalytic theory
**B.** Psychosocial theory
**C.** Behavior modification theory
**D.** Interpersonal theory

**2** The success of a token economy system depends on:

**A.** Consistency of all staff members in rewarding targeted behaviors
**B.** Redemption of tokens for concrete rewards, such as candy, soda, or other snacks
**C.** Setting behavioral goals high enough to motivate the patient
**D.** Flexibility of staff members in allowing for slippage when the patient is having a difficult day

**3** A.'s treatment plan states that he will receive one token for making his bed each morning. After 2 weeks, the nurse reports that A. has not earned any tokens for making his bed. The nurse suggests that:

**A.** The goal remain the same; he will earn a token when he makes his bed
**B.** An attempt to motivate A. should be made by offering him two tokens for making his bed
**C.** The goal should be changed to a one-token penalty when his bed is not made
**D.** The goal should be modified to reflect more attainable goals at this time

**4** A staff member reports that A. may be receiving tokens from other patients who feel sorry for him. Which strategy will control such donations?

**A.** Keep an accurate account of all tokens earned and spent
**B.** Use special, personalized tokens for A.
**C.** Penalize the other patients for giving tokens to A.
**D.** Penalize A. for accepting tokens from others

---

## SITUATION

*D.M., an 8-year-old girl, is admitted to the pediatrics unit after an emergency appendectomy. Parental visits are permitted around the clock, but the nurses are concerned about Mrs. M.'s overprotective behavior. Mrs. M. is almost constantly at her daughter's side, feeding her, bathing her, and talking baby talk to her. She refuses to let D. walk and keeps her in bed to rest and regain her strength.*

*Questions 5 to 7 refer to this situation.*

---

**5** D. has a slightly elevated temperature, and the nurse notes some lung congestion. The best approach to enlist Mrs. M.'s cooperation in D.'s ambulation is to say:

**A.** "You are not helping D. get better by keeping her in bed. She needs to move around to clear her lungs"
**B.** "The physician has told you that D. needs to walk around and get some exercise. Don't you want her to get better?"
**C.** "I want D. to get out of bed at least three times today. Will you help me?"
**D.** "D. needs to move around more because her lungs are getting congested. Let's walk her down the hall and back"

**6** Mrs. M. does not allow D. to do anything for herself. When Mr. M. visits, staff members overhear the parents arguing about Mrs. M.'s babying behavior. Mr. M. asks the nurse if this behavior is normal. How should the nurse respond?

**A.** "Of course it's normal. Your daughter had emergency surgery, and your wife is anxious"
**B.** "I wouldn't be too concerned at this point. Your wife is in a crisis right now"
**C.** "I'd like to learn more about how your wife cares for D. at home"
**D.** "Do *you* think it's normal to be so overprotective?"

**7** Mr. M. asks the nurse to speak with his wife about her overprotectiveness. He says that he has tried everything and that his wife refuses to change. The most appropriate intervention is to:

**A.** Talk to Mrs. M. about her parenting behaviors
**B.** Provide Mr. M. with a referral for family therapy
**C.** Suggest that Mr. M. discuss the problem with D.'s physician
**D.** Ask D. about her relationship with her parents

*After D. is discharged from the hospital, Mr. and Mrs. M. decide to consult a clinical nurse specialist in family therapy.*

*Questions 8 to 10 continue the situation.*

**8** During their initial visit, Mr. and Mrs. M. are asked to complete a chart of their family relationships and history through several generations. This chart is called:

**A.** A family tree
**B.** A genogram
**C.** A sociogram
**D.** Mapping

**9** The nurse therapist will use the chart to identify:

**A.** Multigenerational transmission of presenting signs and symptoms
**B.** Signs and symptoms related to the position of siblings within the family
**C.** Family roles and responsibilities
**D.** Family support systems

**10** When the nurse therapist suggests that Mr. and Mrs. M. bring their daughter with them to the next therapy session, Mrs. M. states, "D. is too young to understand all this. Why should she be involved?" How should the nurse reply?

**A.** "D. may not understand everything we say, but she's part of the problem and should be included"
**B.** "It sounds to me like you are trying to protect D. once again"
**C.** "Perhaps we should ask D. whether or not she wants to be included in our sessions"
**D.** "You've brought up an important issue. Let's discuss why the whole family should attend"

## SITUATION

*F., the nurse-manager in the cardiac clinic, notes that many patients seem confused and overwhelmed by the number of medications prescribed for their heart conditions. She suggests implementing medication management groups. The idea is well received by the treatment team.*

*Questions 11 to 15 refer to this situation.*

**11** F. should begin planning for the groups by carefully assessing:

**A.** The nature of the problems that patients are having with their medications
**B.** Which patients would be interested in joining such a group
**C.** Which staff members are prepared to be leaders or coleaders of the groups
**D.** The best time of day to offer such groups

**12** F. consults the hospital's clinical nurse specialist in psychiatric nursing about group size. The nurse specialist will most likely say that the optimal number of patients in each group is:

**A.** 5
**B.** 10
**C.** 20
**D.** Unlimited

**13** The nurse specialist recommends forming three medication management groups, with F. as leader and another nurse as coleader. Each group meets once a week for 30 minutes in 4-week cycles. What is the best approach to establishing membership in each group?

**A.** Require all cardiac clinic patients to attend
**B.** Assign patients to groups that are offered on their clinic visit days
**C.** Permit patients to join any group or attend any session
**D.** Screen patients, and explain the group's goals and purposes to them

**14** F. and her coleader plan to meet weekly with the clinical nurse specialist for supervision and review of group progress. To facilitate these sessions, the nurse specialist should:

**A.** Ask the leader and coleader to keep a log or journal of each group session
**B.** Review each group member's chart weekly
**C.** Ask the patients how they feel about the group and its progress
**D.** Meet with the leader and coleader separately for supervision

**15** During the group sessions, F. identifies several patients who demonstrate anxiety, ineffective coping, and hopelessness related to the impact of adjusting to a serious cardiac illness. The most beneficial form of group therapy for these patients is likely to be led by:

**A.** F. and another nurse
**B.** A psychiatric clinical nurse specialist
**C.** A cardiology resident
**D.** Other cardiac patients who have coped successfully with similar problems

### SITUATION

*T., a 44-year-old married woman with one son, was referred to the mental health clinic by her family physician after he ruled out any physical basis for her complaints of insomnia, anxiety, fatigue, and loss of interest in her usual activities. On arrival at the clinic, T. states that her symptoms have increased over the last few weeks to the point that she feels "too tired" most of the time to take care of her home or leave the house.*

*Questions 16 to 23 refer to this situation.*

**16** During the initial assessment, the nurse suspects that T. may be having a situational crisis. Which question is most effective in beginning to explore this possibility?

**A.** "What has changed in your life recently?"
**B.** "Do you think your symptoms are related to a recent event in your life?"
**C.** "What do you think is causing your symptoms?"
**D.** "Tell me all about yourself"

**17** T. relates that her father died 7 years ago and that her mother is extremely lonely and misses her father very much. While listening to T., the nurse should further assess for:

**A.** The patient's feelings about her mother
**B.** The patient's feelings about her father
**C.** Any recent losses in the patient's life
**D.** The patient's relationships with relatives and friends

**18** During the assessment interview, T. reveals that her only son moved to another state 2 months ago and that her husband has been traveling frequently on business lately. The nurse inquires about the patient's close relatives and friends. These inquiries should be directed at:

**A.** Encouraging the patient to form closer relationships with others to replace those with her son and husband
**B.** Identifying the patient's available support systems
**C.** Helping the patient to realize she is not alone
**D.** Helping the paitient to develop new coping mechanisms

**19** The treatment team determines that T. is in a situational crisis. Which nursing diagnostic category is most applicable at this time?

A. Dysfunctional grieving
B. Altered thought processes
C. Adjustment disorder
D. Ineffective individual coping

**20** All of the following therapeutic approaches are appropriate for counseling T. *except:*

A. Ventilation
B. Clarification
C. Support of defenses
D. Interpretation

**21** The nurse's role in crisis therapy should be:

A. Nondirective and passive
B. Firm and confrontational
C. Active and directive
D. Calm and nonexpressive

**22** The best indicator that crisis counseling has been effective is T.'s:

A. Working through her feelings of loss over her father's death
B. Developing a closer relationship with her mother
C. Resuming her precrisis routines and activities
D. Visiting her son for several weeks

**23** What is the usual length of time contracted for crisis counseling?

A. 1 to 2 weeks
B. 6 to 8 weeks
C. 3 to 6 months
D. As long as services are necessary

---

## SITUATION

*B.H., age 4, is admitted to the pediatrics unit for treatment of a fractured left humerus and dislocated shoulder. B.'s parents state that he fell down the basement steps. The physical examination reveals multiple bruises on his back, buttocks, arms, and legs and several old fractures of the arm and ribs. A report of suspected child abuse is filed as required by state law, and B. is admitted for further evaluation and treatment.*

*Questions 24 to 27 refer to this situation.*

## 24 The nurse working with B. and his parents should begin by:

**A.** Identifying her feelings and controlling her responses to the suspected child abuse
**B.** Limiting her interaction with B.'s parents until the authorities have spoken with them
**C.** Prohibiting visits by the parents until the suspected child abuse is disproved
**D.** Asking B. whether he wants his parents to visit

## 25 Mrs. H. appears angry and upset by the investigation of B.'s injuries. She yells at the nurse, "He's just a clumsy child. He's always falling or tripping over something. You know how some kids are." Which response by the nurse is most appropriate?

**A.** "I realize this investigation is upsetting you. If what you say is really the case, I'm sure the social worker will find out"
**B.** "I understand this is a difficult time for you. We are required by law to report injuries such as B.'s for further investigation"
**C.** "You sound very defensive. What are you afraid of? Have you been investigated before?"
**D.** "I can't believe that all of B.'s injuries are the result of clumsiness. What really happened?"

## 26 B. remains withdrawn and talks very little. When the nurse gives him some paper and crayons, he draws busily most of the day. Which action should the nurse take regarding B.'s drawings?

**A.** Take several of the drawings from B.'s room to the child psychologist for analysis of their meaning
**B.** Encourage B. to talk about his drawings, asking as many questions as he will tolerate
**C.** Ask B. which drawings represent his family and how his family gets along
**D.** Encourage B. to talk about his feelings, but do not probe if he does not want to talk

**27** Mrs. H. admits that Mr. H. has been abusing her and B. during periods of heavy drinking. Which therapeutic strategy is most helpful for a child such as B.?

A. Play therapy
B. Role playing
C. Group sessions
D. Al-Anon referral

## Answer sheet

|    | A | B | C | D |
|----|---|---|---|---|
| 1  | ○ | ○ | ○ | ○ |
| 2  | ○ | ○ | ○ | ○ |
| 3  | ○ | ○ | ○ | ○ |
| 4  | ○ | ○ | ○ | ○ |
| 5  | ○ | ○ | ○ | ○ |
| 6  | ○ | ○ | ○ | ○ |
| 7  | ○ | ○ | ○ | ○ |
| 8  | ○ | ○ | ○ | ○ |
| 9  | ○ | ○ | ○ | ○ |
| 10 | ○ | ○ | ○ | ○ |
| 11 | ○ | ○ | ○ | ○ |
| 12 | ○ | ○ | ○ | ○ |
| 13 | ○ | ○ | ○ | ○ |
| 14 | ○ | ○ | ○ | ○ |
| 15 | ○ | ○ | ○ | ○ |
| 16 | ○ | ○ | ○ | ○ |
| 17 | ○ | ○ | ○ | ○ |
| 18 | ○ | ○ | ○ | ○ |
| 19 | ○ | ○ | ○ | ○ |
| 20 | ○ | ○ | ○ | ○ |
| 21 | ○ | ○ | ○ | ○ |
| 22 | ○ | ○ | ○ | ○ |
| 23 | ○ | ○ | ○ | ○ |
| 24 | ○ | ○ | ○ | ○ |
| 25 | ○ | ○ | ○ | ○ |
| 26 | ○ | ○ | ○ | ○ |
| 27 | ○ | ○ | ○ | ○ |

## Answers and rationales

**1** Correct answer—**C**

A token economy system uses the principle of reward from the behavior modification theory. Tokens are used to reinforce desired behaviors based on the belief that all behavior is learned. The psychoanalytic theory, which focuses on understanding the unconscious psyche, and the psychosocial and interpersonal theories, which focus on underlying personality development, are not based on reward systems.

**2** Correct answer—**A**

The success of a token economy depends on the full cooperation and coordination of the staff members. Behaviorists have found that consistent rewards produce desired outcomes. All staff members must be knowledgeable about the treatment plan and consistently reward the patient's performance of targeted behaviors. Inconsistent rewards and flexibility are countertherapeutic and encourage manipulation, resistance, and noncompliance. Tokens should be redeemable for items desired by a particular patient. Although food can be used, free time, walks, library privileges, and especially praise are better reinforcers than tangible items, particularly for a teenage patient. Even though the ultimate goal of behavior modification may be extinction (stoppage) of a behavior, beginning goals should be set at a level low enough so that the patient can successfully meet the goal at least part of the time and receive a reinforcer. If this does not occur, the patient will become frustrated and stop trying to change his behavior.

**3** Correct answer—**D**

Goals should be realistic and attainable by the patient. Initial goals may be set rather low to motivate the patient and allow him to attain some success; lack of success can frustrate and discourage the patient. Goals should be reassessed regularly for their appropriateness. In this case, A. has made no progress after 2 weeks, so his situation should be reevaluated. The reinforcers chosen may not mean enough to A. to motivate him to make his bed; new reinforcers may be necessary. Raising the stakes by offering more tokens for a behavior that has not been attained can lead to manipulation of staff members rather than motivation of the patient. Negative reinforcement usually is reserved to discourage maladaptive behaviors, such as fighting, acting out sexually, or cursing. Rewards are given for desired behaviors, not to penalize patients for nonperformance.

## 4 Correct answer—B

A simple, nonpunitive way to end the donations is to reward A. with personalized tokens. He must then redeem his own special tokens, enabling staff members to monitor his behavior. Keeping track of tokens earned and spent by all patients can be an effective way to monitor progress but is a formidable task. Because staff members should encourage positive, helping relationships among patients, penalizing patients for giving or receiving tokens may be misunderstood or misinterpreted.

## 5 Correct answer—D

The nurse can enlist Mrs. M.'s cooperation by teaching her that inactivity is causing her daughter's lung congestion and by assertively telling her what needs to be done. The nurse's remarks should be made in a positive, firm, but nonjudgmental tone. Accusatory responses such as "You're not helping D..." and "Don't you want her to get better?" are likely to be met with defensiveness, not cooperation. These remarks also may shift the focus of the discussion to the mother's behavior rather than that of walking D. Asking for Mrs. M.'s help without restating why it is important does not take advantage of the teaching opportunity presented.

## 6 Correct answer—C

The nurse is presented with an opportunity to further assess Mrs. M.'s parenting behaviors. To determine whether her behavior is a result of the crisis or evidence of more long-standing family dysfunction, the nurse should seek additional data about how Mrs. M. cares for D. at home. Offering false reassurance by telling Mr. M. that his wife's behavior is normal or that he should not worry about it without further exploring his perception of the event denies his feelings and is nontherapeutic. Asking Mr. M if he thinks the behavior is normal puts him in an awkward position because he must then take a stand on whether his wife overprotects his child. A more effective approach is to ask Mr. M. how he feels about the behavior, which allows him to express his feelings and provides the nurse with more assessment data.

**7** Correct answer—**B**

The most appropriate nursing action in this situation is to provide Mr. M. with a referral for family therapy. This decision recognizes that family therapy is a specialized skill requiring careful assessment and analysis and much advanced preparation. Discussing Mrs. M.'s parenting behavior or interviewing D. about her family would serve no purpose unless the nurse is prepared to address the problem in ongoing therapy. Suggesting that Mr. M. discuss the problem with the physician is nontherapeutic because it avoids answering the question directly.

**8** Correct answer—**B**

A genogram is a drawing that charts three or more family generations. It identifies family members, dates of birth, occupations, illnesses, significant life events, and relationships. A family tree displays family members and their dates of birth and death but does not usually detail the other areas mentioned. A sociogram is a diagram that helps identify the frequency and direction of messages and communications patterns (how messages are relayed and to whom) between members of a group or family. The therapist uses the sociogram to assess and evaluate these communications patterns. Family mapping is used by a structural family therapist to assess family system characteristics, such as clear, diffuse, or rigid boundaries; subsystems; and conflicts. Boundaries are the rules defining who participates in which subsystem. Family subsystems consist of individuals, pairs, or groups that form as a result of commonalities such as sex, generation, function, or interest. Interventions are directed toward restructuring the family organization and relationships.

**9** Correct answer—**A**

The purpose of the genogram is to help the family therapist identify patterns of multigenerational transmission of presenting signs and symptoms. Therapists who follow a systems theory framework believe that signs and symptoms have their roots in earlier generations. A family genogram often can identify patterns that on the surface appear to be isolated in the family seeking treatment. Some family therapists believe that the gender and position of siblings—for example, oldest daughter or youngest son—determine personality characteristics that have an impact on relationships with others and adjustments in later life. These therapists focus on the ranking of individuals within the family and are not concerned with a more comprehensive genogram. Neither family roles and responsibilities nor family support systems are designated by the genogram.

## 10 Correct answer—D

In responding to Mrs. M., the nurse should attempt to foster trust and cooperation while helping her understand the importance of each member's participation in the family sessions. Showing acceptance of Mrs. M.'s concern by acknowledging "You have brought up an important issue..." allows the matter to be discussed without placing undue focus on D. or Mrs. M. Attacking Mrs. M.'s protectiveness or putting D. in a position against her mother is not helpful.

## 11 Correct answer—A

When planning groups, the nurse must begin by assessing the patients' needs and resources. Ascertaining the nature of the patients' medication problems is crucial. Once this is accomplished, the nurse can select the leaders and coleaders who are best able to meet the identified patient needs. Establishing the level of patient interest in a group and determining the best time to meet are part of later planning.

## 12 Correct answer—B

Although there is no hard and fast agreement, 10 patients usually is considered an ideal size for a therapeutic group. A group of this size permits opportunities for maximum therapeutic exchange and participation. With 5 or fewer members, participation often is inhibited by self-consciousness. In groups of more than 15 members, overall participation may be inhibited by the formation of smaller patient subgroups. Permitting an unlimited number of members in a group is unwise. Part of the therapeutic benefit is lost if there is no consistency of membership or if the group becomes too large to permit therapeutic interaction.

## 13 Correct answer—D

Group leaders should meet before the group sessions to screen and orient prospective members. At this time, the leader can determine a patient's appropriateness for the group—for example, a patient with a serious hearing problem may benefit more from an individual approach. The screening period also provides the leaders with an opportunity to explain the purpose and goals of the group and to clarify patient expectations. Requiring or assigning patients to groups limits their participation in treatment planning and may result in inappropriate group membership that could be nontherapeutic for other patients. Because consistent group membership encourages attainment of the therapeutic goals, planned patient selection is important.

## 14 Correct answer—A

Using a log or journal to follow and review group progress is an important supervisory aid. The log should document group themes, individual patient responses, and interventions and their effect. The coleader can keep the log during the group meeting or write it as soon as possible after the session ends. The leaders and supervisor can use the log to review group progress and to analyze interventions and strategies. (Other effective methods of tracking group sessions include audiotaping, audiovisual recording, and inviting outsiders to record their observations; however, these methods usually require the patient's consent.) Although patients' records and interviews are a useful part of the group's overall evaluation and effectiveness, they are not helpful in reviewing group progress during supervisory sessions; supervisory sessions should focus on the group leaders and their feelings about the progress of sessions. Having the leader and coleader attend supervisory sessions together allows them to discuss their perceptions of events and enables the supervisor to pursue conflicting statements while the leaders are together.

## 15 Correct answer—B

The psychiatric clinical nurse specialist is an appropriate leader for group therapy with cardiac patients who demonstrate anxiety, ineffective individual coping, and hopelessness. A psychiatric clinical nurse specialist with a master's degree who has been supervised in group therapy has the knowledge and experience necessary for this level of nursing intervention. F., as nurse-manager, might be asked to participate as a coleader but does not have the expertise to lead on her own. A cardiology resident has expertise in medical management but not in group therapy. After the patients have been assisted to develop more effective coping skills, a self-help group composed of other cardiac patients is a means of maintaining these skills.

**16** Correct answer—**A**

Crisis intervention focuses on identifying and solving the patient's immediate presenting problem. By asking about recent changes in the patient's life, the nurse tries to identify factors related to the problem. It is too early in the therapeutic relationship to ask the patient to link her present symptoms to recent life changes. Such analysis needs further exploration and should be based on trust established in the nurse-patient relationship. Because the patient is seeking an answer to her problem, asking her to identify what is causing the symptoms is not helpful. Complete diagnostic assessments typically include extensive explorations of the past and are not done in crisis intervention.

**17** Correct answer—**C**

Identifying underlying themes is an important part of the assessment process in crisis intervention. In this situation, the nurse identifies a theme of loss or abandonment and seeks further clues to recent losses that may have activated the patient's anxiety. The patient's feelings about her mother and father are less important than recent events and her response to them. Once the stressors and the patient's needs are identified, the nurse can assist the patient in identifying positive relationships with friends and relatives.

**18** Correct answer—**B**

During a crisis, a patient typically has difficulty dealing realistically with events, plans, and decisions. Identifying available support networks is an essential part of crisis intervention. The nurse tries to foster adaptive coping and encourage the use of available support systems to help the patient reestablish equilibrium. The nurse should never imply that relationships are replaceable, which belittles the patient's feelings. The nurse may find that the patient has no readily available support system. In this case, the nurse should direct the patient to a crisis group that can provide the needed support. Developing new coping mechanisms is not a primary goal of crisis intervention, which focuses on short-term solutions and is directed toward supporting previous healthy coping mechanisms. Some patients, however, do develop new coping mechanisms in times of crisis.

**19** Correct answer—**D**

The most appropriate nursing diagnostic category for T. is *Ineffective individual coping*. In a crisis, a patient's coping skills are compromised or overwhelmed and become ineffective; equilibrium is typically upset by external events, such as T.'s son moving away and her husband's increased travel. Because the onset of symptoms is clearly related to these events and not to her father's death, the nursing diagnostic category of *Dysfunctional grieving* is unsupported. No evidence supports the diagnostic category of *Altered thought processes,* and *Adjustment disorder* is a medical diagnosis, not a nursing diagnostic category.

**20** Correct answer—**D**

The therapeutic technique of interpretation rarely is used in crisis counseling. Interpretation, which is directed at helping a patient link unconscious factors with present behaviors, is more appropriate in long-term therapy. Ventilation encourages the patient to talk about pent-up feelings to relieve tension. Clarification, a process of verbalizing relationships between events, helps the patient link events in a crisis and understand their relationship; if the patient cannot see the relationships, the nurse may need to point them out. Crisis intervention seeks to support healthy, adaptive defenses rather than develop new ones.

**21** Correct answer—**C**

Because crisis intervention aims for quick resolution of a patient's immediate problem, the nurse must take an active and directive role in this treatment intervention. By using creativity and remaining flexible and open to various therapeutic approaches, the nurse can actively guide the patient through her crisis. A nondirective, passive approach is inappropriate because it fails to recognize that a patient in crisis is in turmoil and needs the direction of others. Being firm may be necessary; however, being confrontational is unwise because it can exacerbate the patient's anxiety. Although remaining calm is an asset, being nonexpressive is nontherapeutic.

**22** Correct answer—**C**

The goal of crisis intervention is to help the patient return to at least her precrisis level of functioning. Resuming routines and activities performed before the crisis is positive evidence of this goal. Resolving long-term issues with continued growth in such areas as relationships with family members is best accomplished by long-term counseling.

## 23 Correct answer—B

Crisis counseling is a short-term approach that usually lasts 6 to 8 weeks, the time during which a crisis is considered acute. Crises are believed to be self-limiting and usually abate within 8 weeks. Situations that are not alleviated within this time are appropriate for long-term counseling or psychotherapy and are not considered crises.

## 24 Correct answer—A

The nurse working with cases of child abuse or other family violence must begin by identifying and examining her own feelings toward such violence. Feelings of anger, disgust, fear, or intimidation must be recognized and controlled for the nurse to intervene effectively. Negative and hostile reactions are likely to intensify maladaptive responses. Instead of avoiding B.'s parents, the nurse should continue to assess their interactions with B. and each other. If B.'s parents pose a significant threat to his physical or psychological safety, appropriate steps should be taken to prevent parental visits. However, B. should not be asked to make a decision regarding parental visitation; asking him whether he wants his parents to visit would be too stressful.

## 25 Correct answer—B

The nurse should respond using emphatic assertion. By acknowledging Mrs. H.'s feelings and stating that the hospital is required to report injuries such as B.'s, the nurse avoids criticizing or rejecting Mrs. H. Statements such as "If that is really the case...," "You sound defensive...," and "I really can't believe..." are judgmental and alienating. Whether or not the child abuse is confirmed, the nurse must foster a therapeutic relationship with the family to intervene effectively.

## 26 Correct answer—D

The nurse should encourage B. to discuss his feelings but should avoid probing him to talk about subjects he wishes to avoid. The goal of therapy is to help the child talk about and deal with the more intense feelings he may be experiencing. Psychiatric staff members will be interested in B.'s drawings, but the nurse should not take the drawings from his room without his consent. Although art therapy requires special training, the nurse can use drawings to encourage nonverbal expression of feelings by both children and adults.

## 27 Correct answer—A

Play therapy is one of the most common and effective strategies used to treat children younger than age 5. Abused children such as B. use play to act out family conflicts, express feelings, and learn behaviors to help protect themselves. Older children who are more verbal and have greater cognitive skills can benefit from such strategies as role playing (acting out situations), group therapy, and Al-Anon (support groups for family and friends of alcoholics).

# CHAPTER 3

# Anxiety Disorders

# Questions

## SITUATION

*T. is the nurse-manager of an oncology unit on the 18th floor of a large urban medical center. Recently, she has been increasingly afraid of riding in the elevator. This morning, she experienced shortness of breath, palpitations, dizziness, and trembling while in the elevator. T. was examined by an emergency department physician, who could find no physiologic basis for her symptoms.*

*Questions 1 to 4 refer to this situation.*

**1** Based on the above findings, T. is most likely suffering from:

**A.** Dissociative disorder
**B.** Phobic disorder
**C.** Obsessive-compulsive disorder
**D.** Somatization disorder

**2** T. begins outpatient counseling sessions with a psychiatric clinical nurse specialist. Which nursing intervention would be most helpful in reducing T.'s anxiety level?

**A.** Psychoanalytically oriented psychotherapy
**B.** Group psychotherapy
**C.** Systematic desensitization
**D.** Referral for evaluation for electroconvulsive therapy

**3** An anxious patient like T. also may benefit greatly from:

**A.** Muscle relaxation
**B.** Psychodrama
**C.** Confrontation
**D.** Biofeedback

**4** Because of the severity of T.'s anxiety, the nurse refers her to a psychiatrist for medication evaluation. Which psychotropic drug regimen is most likely to be prescribed on a short-term basis?

**A.** Diazepam (Valium) 5 mg orally three times a day
**B.** Benztropine mesylate (Cogentin) 2 mg orally twice a day
**C.** Chlorpromazine hydrochloride (Thorazine) 25 mg orally three times a day
**D.** Thioridazine hydrochloride (Mellaril) 100 mg orally four times a day

---

### SITUATION

*B., age 45, is admitted to a psychiatric inpatient unit for treatment of severe obsessive-compulsive disorder.*

*Questions 5 to 9 refer to this situation.*

---

**5** B. has a compulsive bedtime ritual that includes making and remaking his bed 26 times before he can retire. Occasionally, he does not get to bed until 3:00 a.m. Which nursing intervention is most helpful?

**A.** Discussing the ridiculousness of his repetitive behavior
**B.** Taking turns making and remaking the bed with B. to conserve his energy and allow him to retire sooner
**C.** Prohibiting Mr. B. from carrying out his bedtime ritual
**D.** Suggesting that he begin his ritual earlier in the evening so he can retire by 11:30 p.m.

---

**6** Besides performing his nighttime ritual, B. has recently begun a morning bed-making ritual. To help B. limit and potentially alter this maladaptive behavior, all of the following nursing interventions are therapeutic *except:*

**A.** Having B. engage in constructive activities that leave less time for compulsive behaviors
**B.** Verbalizing tactful, mild disapproval of his behavior
**C.** Providing positive reinforcement of nonritualistic behavior
**D.** Offering reflective feedback, such as "I see you have remade your bed many times. You must be exhausted"

---

**7** The nurse must recognize that obsessive-compulsive rituals are an attempt to:

**A.** Increase self-esteem
**B.** Control others
**C.** Express anxiety
**D.** Avoid severe anxiety

---

**8** An appropriately stated short-term goal for this patient is that after 1 week, B. will:

**A.** Demonstrate decreased anxiety
**B.** Participate in a daily exercise group
**C.** Identify the underlying reasons for his rituals
**D.** State that his rituals are irrational

**9** The psychiatrist orders lorazepam (Ativan) 1 mg orally three times a day. While B. is taking this medication, the nurse should remind him to:

**A.** Avoid caffeine
**B.** Avoid aged cheeses
**C.** Stay out of the sun
**D.** Maintain an adequate salt intake

---

## SITUATION

*W., a 20-year-old college junior, is admitted to a medical-surgical unit in a small community hospital after she has a sudden onset of paralysis in both legs. Extensive examination and testing reveal no physical basis for the paralysis. The medical diagnosis is conversion disorder.*

*Questions 10 to 12 refer to this situation.*

**10** The nurse plans interventions for W. based on which correct statement about conversion disorder?

**A.** The symptoms are a conscious attempt to control others in the environment
**B.** The patient will exhibit a high level of anxiety in response to the conversion symptom
**C.** The conversion symptom typically has some symbolic meaning for the patient
**D.** The patient will respond positively to confrontational approaches by the nurse

**11** W. reveals that her boyfriend has been pressuring her to have sex with him. She says, "I love him, but I'm frightened about getting pregnant or getting some disease like AIDS. What should I do?" The nurse's best response would be:

**A.** "There are ways to protect yourself against pregnancy and sexually transmitted diseases. I can refer you to the clinic if you like"
**B.** "You shouldn't let anyone pressure you into sex. Perhaps he doesn't care about you as much as you think he does"
**C.** "It sounds like this problem may be related to your paralysis"
**D.** "Your concerns are realistic. How do you feel about being pressured by your boyfriend?"

**12** During her hospitalization, W. develops insight into her response to threatening situations. When she is discharged, she plans to continue psychotherapy that will focus on:

**A.** Preventing further incidents of paralysis
**B.** Learning new strategies for dealing with stress and conflict
**C.** Breaking off her stress-inducing relationship with her boyfriend
**D.** Developing a healthier attitude toward her sexuality

---

## SITUATION

*S., a 19-year-old college sophomore, makes an appointment at the college health service, where he tells the nurse that he recently has been having trouble concentrating in class. He reports that his grades have suffered because he has been so "out of it." He forgets to do assignments and cannot remember when tests are scheduled. He also reports insomnia, loss of appetite, headaches, and constant fatigue.*

*Questions 13 to 16 refer to this situation.*

**13** S. says to the nurse, "I don't know what's wrong. Either there's something seriously wrong with me, or I must be going crazy." What would be the best response in this situation?

**A.** "You look healthy to me. I'm sure there is nothing seriously wrong with you"
**B.** "It's best not to jump to conclusions. We'll do some tests that should give us a clearer picture of what the problem is"
**C.** "We have an excellent health service here. Whatever the problem is, we will help you"
**D.** "Tell me more about when you began experiencing these symptoms and feelings"

**14** The results of S.'s physical examination and laboratory tests are negative. Two weeks after his initial visit, S. reports that he continues to suffer from nightmares that cause insomnia. He says, "I don't know what to do. Finals are coming up, and I can't study. I'm so exhausted." Which reply by the nurse is best?

**A.** "You mentioned you are having nightmares. Tell me more about them"
**B.** "I understand your frustration. It's terrible not being able to sleep. I can get you a prescription for sleep medication"
**C.** "Have you talked with your professors? Perhaps if they were aware of your problem, you could get extensions for your work"
**D.** "You're exhausted? In what way?"

**15** S. reveals that he was in an automobile accident during final exam week in his freshman year. Although he suffered only minor cuts and bruises, a young man in the other car was killed. In light of this information, the nurse suspects that S. is experiencing:

**A.** Conversion disorder
**B.** Panic disorder
**C.** Phobic disorder
**D.** Post-traumatic stress disorder

**16** Which therapeutic approach is most effective in helping S.?

**A.** Helping him to relax enough to pass his final exams
**B.** Asking the physician to prescribe an antianxiety medication
**C.** Providing new coping mechanisms
**D.** Strengthening current coping mechanisms

---

### SITUATION

*Y. periodically has panic attacks. These attacks are unpredictable and do not seem to be associated with any specific object or situation.*

*Questions 17 to 19 refer to this situation.*

**17** Y. might experience any of the following symptoms during an acute panic attack *except:*

A. Increased perceptual field
B. Increased blood pressure
C. Decreased blood pressure
D. Impaired attention

**18** Which intervention would be most helpful for Y. when she experiences a panic attack?

A. Encouraging her to identify what precipitated the attack
B. Promoting interaction with others to reduce her anxiety through diversion
C. Staying with her and remaining calm, confident, and reassuring
D. Reducing intolerable stimuli by encouraging her to stay in her room alone until she feels less anxious

**19** Which medications have recently been found helpful in reducing or eliminating panic attacks?

A. Antidepressants
B. Anticholinergics
C. Antipsychotics
D. Mood stabilizers

## SITUATION

*A young man is brought to the local emergency department by the police. He approached a police officer in a large metropolitan bus depot stating, "I don't know who or where I am. I have no identification on me. Can you help me?" The young man appears to be in good physical health and between ages 18 and 22. He is clean and neatly groomed. The physical examination reveals no evidence of trauma or other abnormal findings. Staff members refer to him as X.*

*Questions 20 to 23 refer to this situation.*

**20** In the absence of physical findings to explain X.'s memory loss, the most likely diagnosis is:

**A.** Schizophrenia
**B.** Personality disorder
**C.** Somatoform disorder
**D.** Dissociative disorder

**21** X. is admitted to the psychiatric unit for further evaluation and treatment. He probably will react to his inability to recall his identity by exhibiting:

**A.** Intense preoccupation with discovering who he is
**B.** Depression
**C.** Anger and frustration
**D.** Complacency

**22** In working with X., the nurse should direct her first intervention toward:

**A.** Establishing a climate of trust and acceptance
**B.** Identifying the cause of the patient's memory loss
**C.** Encouraging the patient to remember events leading to the memory loss
**D.** Helping the patient recall his first name

**23** Nursing interventions for X. should be based on the understanding that:

**A.** Once the patient's anxiety is alleviated, his memory will return
**B.** Memory loss usually is precipitated by severe psychologic stress
**C.** The patient could remember his identity if he really wanted to
**D.** The patient probably will regain his memory slowly but have an incomplete recall of immediate events

## SITUATION

*P., a 40-year-old mother of two children ages 6 and 9, is admitted for a surgical biopsy of a suspicious lump in her left breast.*

*Questions 24 to 26 refer to this situation.*

**24** The admitting nurse wants to assess P.'s perceptions about her admission and proposed treatment. Which question is the best way to initiate such a discussion?

**A.** "What has your physician told you about the reason for your admission?"
**B.** "Have you discussed the treatment alternatives available to you if the lump is malignant?"
**C.** "What questions do you have about your admission and treatment?"
**D.** "What is your understanding of the reasons for your admission and the possible courses of treatment?"

**25** P. says to the nurse, "I don't want to be put to sleep for this biopsy. I want to be awake and aware of what's happening. That's the best way to do this, isn't it?" How should the nurse respond?

**A.** "Everyone reacts differently, but I agree with you. I'd want to be awake, too"
**B.** "You will be medicated to help you feel relaxed. I wouldn't worry about it"
**C.** "That's really between you and your surgeon. You'd better discuss this with him"
**D.** "Tell me more about your thoughts on being awake or asleep during the biopsy"

**26** When the nurse comes to take P. to surgery, she finds her tearfully finishing a letter to her children. P. says, "I want to leave this for them in case anything goes wrong today." The nurse's best response would be:

**A.** "In case anything goes wrong? What are your thoughts right now?"
**B.** "I can understand that you're nervous, but this is really a minor procedure. You'll be back in your room before you know it"
**C.** "Try and take a few deep breaths and relax. I have some medication that will help"
**D.** "I'm sure your children know how much you love them. You'll be able to talk to them on the phone in a few hours"

# Answer sheet

A B C D
1 ○○○○
2 ○○○○
3 ○○○○
4 ○○○○
5 ○○○○
6 ○○○○
7 ○○○○
8 ○○○○
9 ○○○○
10 ○○○○
11 ○○○○
12 ○○○○
13 ○○○○
14 ○○○○
15 ○○○○
16 ○○○○
17 ○○○○
18 ○○○○
19 ○○○○
20 ○○○○
21 ○○○○
22 ○○○○
23 ○○○○
24 ○○○○
25 ○○○○
26 ○○○○

## Answers and rationales

**1** Correct answer—**B**

A phobic disorder is characterized by a persistent fear of some object or situation that presents no real danger or that magnifies the danger out of proportion. An example of this disorder is T.'s fear of riding in the elevator. A dissociative disorder occurs when a patient blocks off from consciousness some aspect of his life because of the threat of overwhelming anxiety. Amnesia is an example of dissociative disorder. An obsessive-compulsive disorder is manifested by repetitive thoughts or recurring impulses to perform certain acts—for example, frequent hand washing. A somatization disorder occurs when a patient experiences some physical dysfunctioning resulting from profound anxiety over a repressed drive, such as the sexual drive. An example of this disorder is that of a patient who experiences blindness after becoming aroused by accidentally seeing his sister in the shower.

**2** Correct answer—**C**

Phobias commonly are viewed as learned responses to anxiety that can be unlearned through certain techniques, such as behavior modification. Systematic desensitization, a form of behavior modification, attempts to reduce anxiety and thereby eradicate the patient's phobia through gradual exposure to anxiety-producing stimuli. For example, a patient who is afraid of flying could be desensitized by first viewing pictures of airplanes, then going to the airport, and later just sitting in a plane before attempting to fly. Psychoanalytically oriented therapy also may be effective in this situation because recall of childhood experiences can help the patient clarify and understand her phobia. However, such therapy requires years of treatment. Group psychotherapy, which involves treating patients in groups, could be used as an adjunct treatment to help increase the patient's self-esteem and lower her generalized anxiety. Electroconvulsive therapy, the use of electric current to produce a convulsive seizure, is primarily reserved for patients with severe depression or psychosis who have responded poorly to other treatments. It usually is not indicated for phobic disorders.

**3** Correct answer—**A**

Muscle relaxation techniques—the systematic tensing and relaxing of major muscle groups—decrease anxiety and relax the body. They are an important adjunct to systematic desensitization. Psychodrama is the dramatization of a patient's interactions and problems. Confrontation involves calling attention to discrepancies, such as the inconsistency between a patient's affect and his verbal expressions. Psychodrama and confrontational approaches are primarily used to resolve interpersonal issues. Biofeedback attempts to bring certain autonomic functions, such as heart rate and blood pressure, under voluntary control. Biofeedback training is more useful for reducing stress associated with physiologically based disorders, such as hypertension, asthma, and gastritis.

## 4 Correct answer—A

Diazepam (Valium) is the most appropriate medication for this patient because of its antianxiety properties. Benztropine mesylate (Cogentin) is an antiparkinsonian agent used to control the extrapyramidal side effects of such antipsychotic medications as chlorpromazine hydrochloride (Thorazine) and thioridazine hydrochloride (Mellaril). Chlorpromazine and thioridazine are used to control the severe symptoms (hallucinations, thought disorders, agitation) seen in patients with psychosis.

## 5 Correct answer—D

At present, B. needs this behavioral pattern to keep his anxiety within tolerable bounds. Suggesting that he begin the ritual during free time in the evening sets some limits but allows him to continue performing the behavior. Patients such as B. usually are aware of the irrationality of their actions yet feel unable to stop them. Helping with the ritual is a nontherapeutic reinforcement of the behavior. Attempting to prevent B. from performing his ritual would increase his anxiety and possibly precipitate panic.

## 6 Correct answer—B

Verbalizing even minimal disapproval of B.'s behavior would increase his anxiety and consequently reinforce his need to perform the rituals. Engaging B. in constructive activity provides an outlet for his energy without channeling it into compulsive behavior. Providing positive reinforcement of nonritualistic behavior tends to strengthen these constructive activities. Reflective feedback lets B. know that the nurse recognizes the behavior and understands how tiring it can be.

**7** Correct answer—**D**

Obsessive-compulsive rituals are an attempt to avoid increasing anxiety to a severe level. Although the patient may feel the need to increase his self-esteem, this is not the primary reason for performing obsessive-compulsive rituals. The patient is not attempting to control others because he is anxious and preoccupied with his own behaviors. The patient's ritualistic behavior is not a means of expressing anxiety but a way to avoid it.

**8** Correct answer—**B**

Participating in a daily exercise group refocuses the patient's time toward adaptive activities and may reduce his anxiety. "Demonstrate decreased anxiety" is not stated specifically enough to allow for evaluation. For this goal to be measurable, specific objectives must be stated, such as that B. will verbalize he is feeling less anxious. Insight into the underlying reasons for the rituals takes time to develop and is not a realistic goal after 1 week. A patient with an obsessive-compulsive disorder typically is well aware of the irrationality of the ritual but is unable to stop it.

**9** Correct answer—**A**

Ingesting 500 mg or more of caffeine can significantly alter the anxiolytic effects of lorazepam. Other dietary restrictions are unnecessary. Aged cheeses must be avoided when taking monamine oxidase (MAO) inhibitors. Staying out of the sun or using sunscreens is required when taking phenothiazines. An adequate salt intake is necessary for patients receiving lithium.

**10** Correct answer—**C**

A conversion disorder, sometimes called hysteria, is a type of somatoform disorder in which the patient exhibits a symptom (such as a tic, tremor, or paralysis) that symbolically represents a conflict the patient is experiencing. The manifested symptom is not a conscious attempt to control others. Instead of being anxious, the patient characteristically exhibits indifference to the symptoms. This reaction initially represents an unconscious control of anxiety. Confrontation threatens the patient's defense against anxiety and is therefore nontherapeutic.

## 11 Correct answer—D

Because conversion disorders commonly arise from conflicts and tension associated with sexual drives, W. must be encouraged to explore her concerns about having sex with her boyfriend. The nurse should acknowledge the patient's feelings and encourage her to discuss them. The other options may be helpful, but they do not promote exploration of the realistic aspects of the patient's conflict.

## 12 Correct answer—B

The patient needs to learn new and more adaptive coping strategies, such as talking about her feelings and not denying them, to help her deal with life's many stressors. Paralysis is only a symptom of W.'s underlying problem and would not be the focus of psychotherapy. Unless W. learns to cope with the conflict associated with her sexual drives, her next relationship also will result in stress. Her problem is not her sexuality but the stress associated with it.

## 13 Correct answer—D

The nurse needs to find out more about the onset of the patient's symptoms. To fully assess the patient, she should determine how long the symptoms have been present, when they started, and whether there were any precipitating events, such as a breakup with a girlfriend. Options A and B may be true, but they cut off further exploration of the patient's symptoms. They also may be viewed as false reassurance and an attempt to deny the validity of the patient's feelings. Option C focuses on the health service and not on S.'s problem.

## 14 Correct answer—A

Exploring the content of S.'s nightmares can provide clues to his underlying conflict. For example, a veteran may have recurring nightmares related to his war experiences. Acknowledging the patient's feelings without exploring them further is not enough. Offering sleep medication is inappropriate because this is only a temporary measure; S. should be encouraged to explore the underlying stressors and to find effective ways of coping rather than dismiss his symptoms with medication. Focusing on S.'s exhaustion is not as helpful as exploring its possible causes. Although talking with his professors may help S. to get an extension on his schoolwork, doing so will not address his underlying problems or help him to sleep better.

## 15 Correct answer—D

Post-traumatic stress disorder (PTSD) is a form of anxiety disorder in which an individual relives an extremely stressful experience with accompanying guilt and dysfunction. PTSD can cause a delayed response to a traumatic event—in S.'s case, the fatal automobile accident. In a conversion disorder, the patient's anxiety is temporarily managed by his symptoms, and distress is not apparent. In a panic disorder, the patient typically experiences severe anxiety resulting in feelings of impending death. In a phobic disorder, the patient characteristically experiences fear of an object or situation that presents no real danger.

## 16 Correct answer—C

To deal with his traumatic memories, S. needs to learn new coping strategies—for instance, systematic desensitization. Helping S. to relax enough so that he can pass his final exams may or may not be realistic and is secondary to the overall treatment goals. Medication should be used only if necessary; although drugs can relieve some of the symptoms of anxiety, they do not remove its underlying causes. The inadequacy of S.'s current coping skills has led him to seek help.

## 17 Correct answer—A

Panic is the most severe level of anxiety. During a panic attack, the patient experiences a decrease, not an increase, in perceptual field. She becomes more focused on herself and is less aware of what is happening around her. The patient becomes unable to process information from her environment. The decreased perceptual field contributes to impaired attention and the inability to concentrate. Increased blood pressure related to stimulation of the sympathetic nervous system or decreased blood pressure related to stimulation of the parasympathetic nervous system can also occur.

## 18 Correct answer—C

A panic-stricken patient requires the assistance of a calm person who can provide support and direction. This is particularly important because the patient already feels frightened and out of control.

Having someone remain with the patient prevents feelings of isolation and desertion. Encouraging the patient to identify what precipitated the attack is futile because the patient is too anxious to focus on precipitating factors. When the patient feels extremely anxious, interaction with others is difficult. Reducing stimuli can be helpful, but having the patient stay alone may increase her anxiety.

## 19 Correct answer—A

Tricyclic and MAO inhibitor antidepressants have been found effective in treating patients with panic attacks. Why these drugs control the attacks is not clearly understood. Anticholinergic agents, which are smooth-muscle relaxants, help relieve the physical symptoms of anxiety but do not relieve the anxiety itself. Patients who experience panic attacks are not psychotic, so antipsychotic drugs are inappropriate. Mood stabilizers are not indicated because mood changes are not usually associated with panic attacks.

## 20 Correct answer—D

The patient in this situation is probably suffering from a dissociative disorder, which is characterized by a temporary alteration in consciousness, identity, or motor behavior in response to stress, anxiety, or perceived danger. Psychogenic amnesia, a sudden inability to recall extensive amounts of personal data because of a physical or psychological trauma, is an example of this type of disorder. Schizophrenia, a type of psychosis in which the patient responds to overwhelming anxiety through a disintegration of ego functioning, is characterized by impaired communication and loss of contact with reality. X. shows no evidence of thought disorder or other psychotic symptoms, so a diagnosis of schizophrenia is not indicated. A personality disorder typically originates within the character structure of the individual and is evidenced by a lifelong pattern of maladaptive behavior rather than one of acute onset. Examples include such conditions as antisocial and borderline personality. A somatoform disorder is characterized by multiple physiological complaints or symptoms having no organic basis.

## 21 Correct answer—D

Because a patient with psychogenic amnesia is successfully blocking a traumatic or severe anxiety-producing event, he will probably react to his inability to recall his identity with complacency. He will not have an intense desire to discover who he is because learning his identity would force him to remember the event and confront the anxiety he so fears. For the same reason, X. will not exhibit depression or anger, both of which are associated with anxiety-producing events.

## 22 Correct answer—A

Because the patient is defending himself against severe anxiety, the nurse must first establish a warm, trusting, and accepting climate. After gaining the patient's trust, the nurse can help him learn ways to deal with his anxiety. Prodding X. to recall events or remember his name is not helpful at this time. Identifying the cause of the patient's memory loss may be impossible.

## 23 Correct answer—B

Psychogenic amnesia usually is precipitated by severe psychologic stress that causes the patient to repress (block out) painful events or experiences. Both the stressful event and the anxiety that it produced have been blocked from X.'s memory. Until the stressful event is identified, the accompanying anxiety cannot be alleviated. Forgetting one's identity is an unconscious act, and willing oneself to remember is not enough to be successful. Slow return of memory with impaired recall of the amnesia period is characteristic of memory loss caused by head injury.

## 24 Correct answer—D

By asking the patient to explain her understanding of the situation, the nurse can assess both her knowledge and her emotional reactions. Often, the anxiety produced by being told one might have cancer is so great that the patient cannot absorb further details given by a physician. Asking P. what the physician has said or what questions she might have can be done later to clarify and evaluate her initial responses.

## 25 Correct answer—D

The nurse needs to explore the patient's statement further before responding. The nurse's role is not to agree or disagree with the patient's choices. Telling the patient not to worry about the procedure would be inappropriate; the nurse should explore the patient's concerns, not minimize them. Although the final decision is between the patient and her surgeon, the nurse can help the patient explore and clarify her feelings at this time.

**26** Correct answer—**A**

By acknowledging how the patient feels, the nurse encourages further expression of the patient's thoughts. Minimizing feelings or offering empty reassurance is not empathetic or helpful. Deep breathing or preoperative medications are appropriate after the patient's fears have been expressed and dealt with.

# CHAPTER 4

# Mood Disorders

# Questions

**SITUATION**

*B., age 42, is brought to the hospital by her husband, who reports that she has been neglecting her housework and family responsibilities and eating very little and has not left the house for the past 2 months. She is 5'7" (170 cm) tall and normally weighs 147 lb (66.7 kg), but during the past 8 weeks, she has lost 20 lb (9.1 kg). Mrs. B.'s history reveals that her 7-month-old daughter recently died of sudden infant death syndrome (SIDS). She is admitted to the psychiatric unit with a diagnosis of depression.*

*Questions 1 to 15 refer to this situation.*

**1** Immediately after admission, B. isolates herself in her room. The nurse should approach the patient with the understanding that:

**A.** Depressed patients like B. commonly are suicidal and establishing a trusting relationship is key to preventing suicide
**B.** B. probably believes she is not ill and therefore will not socialize with others at this point
**C.** B. is isolating herself because her family is not available to support her
**D.** B.'s illness and hospitalization for emotional problems have a negative impact on her and her family

**2** The nurse helps B. to settle in. While observing B. unpack, the nurse expects her to exhibit:

**A.** Fast, hurried movements
**B.** Slow, retarded movements
**C.** A desire to initiate a conversation with her roommates
**D.** A desire to unpack and arrange her belongings without assistance

**3**
Early that evening, B. tearfully tells the nurse, "I feel so guilty. I left the window open in my daughter's room. Maybe she got chilled during the night. Perhaps the crib should have been on the other side of the room." How should the nurse respond?
**A.** "You're still young. You and your husband can have another child if you want"
**B.** "I don't think that's what caused your daughter's death. You have other children you should be concerned about"
**C.** "You shouldn't feel guilty, B. Why don't you try to forget about such sad memories"
**D.** "Your daughter died of SIDS, B. It was not your fault"

**4** The following day, the nurse finds B. pacing the hallways, wringing her hands, picking at her hair and skin, and saying, "I don't know what to do. I don't know what to do." The most appropriate nursing action at this time is to:

**A.** Take the patient back to her room and encourage her to rest
**B.** Calmly tell the patient to pull herself together
**C.** Encourage the patient to help water the plants in the dayroom
**D.** Permit the patient to continue her behavior until she feels less anxious

**5** After 1 week, B. states, "Now that my baby is dead and I'm too old to have another one, I don't want to live anymore." The nurse should respond by saying:

**A.** "Life doesn't look very promising to you right now, but let's talk about this"
**B.** "You shouldn't feel so hopeless. Many women are having babies in their forties"
**C.** "I care about you, and I want you to live"
**D.** "What about your husband and other children? Don't you think they need you?"

**6** B. is started on imipramine (Tofranil) 75 mg orally at bedtime. The nurse should tell the patient that:

**A.** The medication may be habit forming, so it will be discontinued as soon as she feels better
**B.** The medication has no serious side effects
**C.** She should avoid eating such foods as aged cheeses, yogurt, and chicken livers while taking the medication
**D.** The medication may initially cause some tiredness, which should become less bothersome over time

**7** The nurse should inform B. that the full therapeutic benefits of imipramine may not take effect for:

**A.** 3 to 7 days
**B.** 2 to 3 weeks
**C.** 3 to 4 weeks
**D.** 2 months or more

**8** B. does not respond to the medication. At a team conference, staff members recommend electroconvulsive therapy (ECT). When should nursing interventions begin?

**A.** As soon as the patient and her family are presented with this treatment alternative
**B.** The night before ECT is scheduled
**C.** Immediately after ECT is administered
**D.** When the patient returns to the unit after ECT therapy

**9** Most people respond emotionally to the thought of electric current passing through their brain. When discussing the subject with the patient, the nurse should:

**A.** Use the term "shock" in a neutral, calm manner
**B.** Refer to the procedure as the patient's "treatment" instead of "shock therapy"
**C.** Refer to it as ECT
**D.** Explain how the convulsions are artificially induced

**10** B. and her husband begin to express concern about the proposed ECT treatment. Which nursing action is most appropriate initally?

**A.** Refer all questions to the physician who will actually administer the ECT treatment
**B.** Listen for misconceptions and clarify any confusing information
**C.** Orient B. and her husband to the ECT unit so they become familiar and comfortable with the surroundings
**D.** Provide B. and her husband with booklets explaining the procedure in simple, understandable terms

**11** By providing B. and her husband with an opportunity to discuss ECT treatment openly and directly, the nurse communicates the idea that:

**A.** ECT should not be feared
**B.** ECT will reverse the depression
**C.** ECT is a positive treatment alternative
**D.** ECT is a safe procedure

**12** B. asks the nurse, "Why do I have to sign a consent form?" Which response is most appropriate?

**A.** "It indicates that you have been fully informed about the procedure and the risks involved"
**B.** "Your physician should have explained this to you yesterday. Didn't he tell you about signing a consent?"
**C.** "It's just a hospital rule. Sign here, please"
**D.** "Most of the medications used can be dangerous. Your consent is required"

**13** When B. returns to her room after awakening from the ECT treatment, the nurse should:

**A.** Place a "No visitors" sign on the door so she can rest undisturbed
**B.** Perform a complete physical assessment
**C.** Orient her to person, place, and time
**D.** Remain with her until all confusion disappears

**14** Which other nursing action should the nurse perform after the patient returns from ECT treatment?

**A.** Take vital signs every 15 minutes for the next 2 hours
**B.** Open all locked closets so the patient can have access to her belongings
**C.** Offer the patient a cigarette if she smokes, to help her relax
**D.** Touch the patient by grasping her hand or massaging her shoulders while talking to her

**15** Which side effects are most common after ECT treatment?

**A.** Headache and dizziness
**B.** Diarrhea and urinary incontinence
**C.** Nausea and vomiting
**D.** Temporary memory loss and confusion

## SITUATION

*C., age 36 and single, is brought to the local psychiatric hospital by her brother, who tells the nurse that she has been involved in a whirlwind of activity that began several months ago and that she seems out of control. She told friends that she was devoting all her time to writing a novel that was nearly complete, but at the same time, she began painting the interior of her seven-room home. When her friends tried to get her to slow down, she increased her activities, taking little time to sleep or eat, and began spending huge amounts of money. Her admission was necessitated when she wrote a check for $500,000, with a bank balance of only $5.*

*At admission, C. is agitated, speaking loudly and challenging other patients. Her admitting diagnosis is bipolar reaction, manic phase.*

*Questions 16 to 23 refer to this situation.*

**16** Which approach would be most therapeutic in working with C.?

**A.** Teaching the patient about banking procedures, then extending this approach to everyday issues
**B.** Confronting the patient about all her inappropriate behavior
**C.** Kindly but firmly guiding the patient into such activities as bathing and eating
**D.** Showing the patient that she is in a controlled environment so that no difficulties arise later

**17** C. lost 15 lb (6.8 kg) last week and now weighs 100 lb (45.4 kg). The nurse formulates a nursing diagnosis based on the diagnostic category *Altered nutrition: less than body requirements.* Which goal is most appropriate initially?

A. The patient will consume an adequate diet
B. The patient will maintain her current weight of 100 lb
C. The patient will gain 1 lb (0.5 kg) per week
D. The patient will remain adequately hydrated

**18** The best approach to meeting C.'s hydration and nutrition needs would be to:

A. Leave finger foods and liquids in her room and let her eat and drink as she moves about
B. Bring her to the dining room and encourage her to sit and eat with calm, quiet companions
C. Explain mealtime routines and allow her to make her own decisions about eating
D. Provide essential nutrition through high-calorie gavage feedings

**19** The physician decides to start C. on lithium (Lithane) therapy. Which of the following best describes her dietary requirements while she is receiving this medication?

A. A high-calorie diet with reduced sodium and adequate fluid intake
B. A regular diet with normal sodium and adequate fluid intake
C. A low-calorie diet with reduced sodium and increased fluid intake
D. A regular diet with reduced sodium and adequate fluid intake

**20** A few days later, C. tells the nurse, "I'm so ashamed of myself. I don't deserve to be here and be taken care of." Which action best demonstrates the nurse's understanding of the patient's needs?

A. Expressing relief that C. has recognized the foolishness of her behavior
B. Calling a team conference to increase protection against possible self-destructive behavior by C.
C. Reporting to staff members that C. appears to be developing insight into her behavior
D. Telling C. that she has done nothing that she should regret

**21** C. would benefit most from which activity during the manic phase of her illness?

A. Playing a game of badminton
B. Attending the unit's weekly bingo game
C. Putting together an intricate puzzle
D. Drawing or painting in her room

**22** One week after C. begins taking lithium, the nurse notes that her serum lithium level is 1 mEq/liter. How should the nurse respond?

A. Call the physician immediately to report the laboratory results
B. Observe the patient closely for signs of lithium toxicity
C. Withhold the next dose and repeat the blood work
D. Continue administering the medication as ordered

**23** Early signs of lithium toxicity include:

A. Fine tremors, nausea, vomiting, and diarrhea
B. Ataxia, confusion, and seizures
C. Elevated white blood cell count and orthostatic hypotension
D. Restlessness, shuffling gait, and involuntary muscle movements

---

### SITUATION

*Two days ago, M. arrived on the psychiatric unit, exhibiting extreme excitement, disorientation, incoherent speech, agitation, frantic, aimless physical activity, and grandiose delusions.*

*Questions 24 to 26 refer to this situation.*

**24** M. is in a manic episode. Which assessment finding is most characteristic of this stage of mania?

A. Mild elation
B. Hypomania
C. Acute elation
D. Delirium

**25** Which nursing diagnostic category would hold the highest priority for M. at this time?

A. Ineffective individual coping
B. Hopelessness
C. Potential for injury
D. Personal identity disturbance

**26** M. is assigned to a private room that is somewhat removed from the nurse's station. The primary reason for this room assignment is to:

A. Decrease environmental stimuli
B. Prevent the patient's excessive activity from disturbing others
C. Deter the patient from interrupting the nurses
D. Provide the patient with a quiet environment for thinking about his problems

## SITUATION

*K. is admitted to the acute psychiatric unit after 2 weeks of increasingly erratic behavior. She has not been sleeping, has lost 8 lb (3.6 kg), and is poorly groomed. She is hyperactive and loudly denies her need for hospitalization.*

*Questions 27 to 30 refer to this situation.*

**27** A priority nursing intervention for K. is to:

A. Provide adequate hygiene
B. Administer sedative medication
C. Decrease environmental stimuli
D. Involve her in unit activities

**28** The physician plans to order lithium carbonate for K. Before beginning the lithium treatment regimen, the nurse performs a physical assessment. She is aware that lithium is contraindicated when a patient exhibits dysfunction of the:

A. Renal system
B. Reproductive system
C. Endocrine system
D. Respiratory system

**29** The physician changes the medication order to lithium carbonate 300 mg four times a day and chlorpromazine (Thorazine) 100 mg four times a day. Which statement best explains the reason for ordering chlorpromazine?

**A.** A lower dose of lithium can be given
**B.** Chlorpromazine helps control the manic symptoms until the lithium takes effect
**C.** Joint administration makes both drugs more effective
**D.** Joint administration decreases the risk of lithium toxicity

**30** After 10 days on the unit, K. can tolerate short periods in the dayroom. One day, the nurse overhears her tell another patient that she is a journalist posing as a patient so that she can gather enough information to write an article about mental hospitals. The nurse should:

**A.** Ignore K.'s delusion
**B.** Confront K.
**C.** Take K. back to her room
**D.** Support K.'s denial of her illness

## Answer sheet

|    | A | B | C | D |
|----|---|---|---|---|
| 1  | ○ | ○ | ○ | ○ |
| 2  | ○ | ○ | ○ | ○ |
| 3  | ○ | ○ | ○ | ○ |
| 4  | ○ | ○ | ○ | ○ |
| 5  | ○ | ○ | ○ | ○ |
| 6  | ○ | ○ | ○ | ○ |
| 7  | ○ | ○ | ○ | ○ |
| 8  | ○ | ○ | ○ | ○ |
| 9  | ○ | ○ | ○ | ○ |
| 10 | ○ | ○ | ○ | ○ |
| 11 | ○ | ○ | ○ | ○ |
| 12 | ○ | ○ | ○ | ○ |
| 13 | ○ | ○ | ○ | ○ |
| 14 | ○ | ○ | ○ | ○ |
| 15 | ○ | ○ | ○ | ○ |
| 16 | ○ | ○ | ○ | ○ |
| 17 | ○ | ○ | ○ | ○ |
| 18 | ○ | ○ | ○ | ○ |
| 19 | ○ | ○ | ○ | ○ |
| 20 | ○ | ○ | ○ | ○ |
| 21 | ○ | ○ | ○ | ○ |
| 22 | ○ | ○ | ○ | ○ |
| 23 | ○ | ○ | ○ | ○ |
| 24 | ○ | ○ | ○ | ○ |
| 25 | ○ | ○ | ○ | ○ |
| 26 | ○ | ○ | ○ | ○ |
| 27 | ○ | ○ | ○ | ○ |
| 28 | ○ | ○ | ○ | ○ |
| 29 | ○ | ○ | ○ | ○ |
| 30 | ○ | ○ | ○ | ○ |

# Answers and rationales

**1** Correct answer—**A**

Preventing suicide takes priority over other needs. Once a trusting relationship is established, B. will more readily discuss her fears. If the patient senses that the nurse is concerned and can be trusted, she will feel less alone and believe that someone understands. The patient's perception of her illness is unknown, as is the level of family support and the impact of her hospitalization. All other needs are secondary to the patient's safety needs at this time.

**2** Correct answer—**B**

The behavior of the depressed patient is typically slow, retarded, and fatiguing. Such a patient also has difficulty interacting, making decisions, and initiating independent actions. Nursing interventions should be planned to assist and support the patient as needed to meet her needs. Although increased activity may be observed in patients with agitated depression (depression with frantic pacing), it is more common in those with mania.

**3** Correct answer—**D**

The nurse should restate and reinforce that the child's death was not B.'s fault, nor was it related to her actions. Sudden infant death syndrome strikes unexpectedly; it has no symptoms or warning signs. Denying the patient's feelings of loss is both nontherapeutic and insensitive.

**4** Correct answer—**C**

A simple task like watering the plants provides a purposeful activity to focus the patient's energy as well as human contact and a sense of accomplishment. By encouraging assistance in this activity, the nurse attempts to increase B.'s self-esteem. Isolating the patient in her room, telling her to pull herself together, and ignoring her distress by not intervening are nontherapeutic approaches.

**5** Correct answer—**A**

Reflecting the patient's feeling by responding "Life doesn't look very promising right now..." validates how the patient feels and encourages her to ventilate further. Although the nurse should let the patient know that she cares and will protect her, such responses as "You shouldn't feel so hopeless," "What about your husband and children," or even simply "I care" deny the patient's feelings, cut her off, and shift the focus to how others feel. The nurse should provide an opportunity for the patient to express her feelings.

## 6 Correct answer—D

Sedation is a common early side effect of the tricyclic antidepressant imipramine (Tofranil) and usually decreases as tolerance develops. Antidepressants are not habit forming; they do not cause physical or psychological dependence. However, after they are taken at high doses for long periods, the dosage should be decreased gradually to avoid mild withdrawal symptoms. Serious side effects, although rare, can occur; they include myocardial infarction, congestive heart failure, and tachycardia. Dietary restrictions, such as avoiding aged cheeses, yogurt, and chicken livers, are necessary for a patient taking monoamine oxidase (MAO) inhibitors, not tricyclic antidepressants.

## 7 Correct answer—C

Antidepressant agents such as imipramine usually produce a noticeable effect in 2 to 3 weeks but do not reach full therapeutic effectiveness until 3 to 4 weeks after initiation of therapy. If no improvement is noted by that time, the medication is considered ineffective and a new drug is tried. The nurse must be sure to teach the patient that the drug's effect will occur gradually and that discontinuing it before peak effectiveness is achieved will render the drug useless. She also must encourage and support the patient during this time because the depressed patient may expect more immediate relief from the medication.

## 8 Correct answer—A

The nurse is responsible for assessing the patient's and family members' response to electroconvulsive therapy (ECT) and for providing opportunities for communication regarding their feelings and concerns as soon as the treatment is proposed. ECT is rarely an initial treatment for depression; it is used when a patient responds poorly to medication. It involves inducing a seizure in the patient by passing electric current through the brain (seizures are thought to produce changes in neurotransmitters and receptor sites similar to those produced by antidepressant medications). Before the treatment, the patient is given a short-acting barbiturate to induce anesthesia. After the procedure, the patient typically awakens quickly but remains confused and light-headed, necessitating close nursing supervision until these effects subside. Although the patient is not aware of the actual seizure, she may be upset by the temporary memory loss; therefore, a supportive nursing approach is essential. Nurșing interventions continue before, during, and after each ECT treatment.

## 9 Correct answer—**B**

To emphasize the therapeutic value of ECT, the nurse should refer to it as the patient's "treatment." Although "ECT" is medically correct terminology, this term should not be used unless the patient is familiar and comfortable with it; referring to the procedure as ECT may cause the patient to focus on the disturbing elements of this treatment. Such terms as "convulsions" and "shock" tend to increase a patient's anxiety and should therefore be avoided.

## 10 Correct answer—**B**

Although controversial, ECT is an effective treatment for depression. Many people have negative images about ECT treatment that may have arisen from reading about ECT or watching movies in which it is portrayed as barbaric or inhumane. The nurse can be most helpful by listening carefully to the patient to assess her fears and needs and then determining how to intervene. If needed, the patient then can be referred to the physician, oriented to the area, or given booklets explaining the procedure. The patient has the right to make an informed consent and, if competent, to refuse any treatment, including ECT.

## 11 Correct answer—**C**

Openly discussing the proposed ECT treatment places an appropriate emphasis on accepting the therapeutic value of the procedure. The nurse should be supportive while realistically discussing the treatment outcomes, the patient's fears, and any potential untoward effects of the ECT treatment. Because ECT involves the use of an anesthetic and the passing of an electric current through the brain, fear is a normal, expected response. Although ECT has proved to be an effective treatment for lessening the degree of depression, it is not guaranteed to reverse the depression. In the role of patient advocate, the nurse cannot imply that there are no safety concerns. Although uncommon, such adverse effects as permanent memory loss, periodic hypertension, and stroke can occur.

## 12 Correct answer—A

The nurse should restate the purpose of signing a consent form, which is to ensure that the patient has been informed of the benefits and risks of the procedure. The patient probably is anxious and may have forgotten what she was told earlier. The consent form is an important legal document, and the patient has the right to know its purpose; even if the physician explained the procedure, the patient must understand what she is signing before she signs it. The patient's signature indicates awareness and understanding, not just compliance with hospital policy. Because ECT involves risks other than those associated with medication, these risks must be fully understood.

## 13 Correct answer—C

A patient returning from ECT treatment typically is confused and disoriented. The nurse's task is to reassure the patient by orienting her to person, place, and time. Although the patient will be tired, she can receive visitors. A complete physical assessment is not needed after an ECT treatment. The nurse cannot remain with the patient until all confusion disappears because this may take several days.

## 14 Correct answer—D

Touch reinforces verbal encouragement, demonstrates caring, strengthens interactions, and establishes the nurse's presence and availability. Vital signs are monitored in the recovery room until the patient is stable. Until the patient is fully alert and ambulatory, the nurse should keep the closets locked to protect the patient's valuables. The patient should not be permitted to smoke until she can safely go to a smoking area.

## 15 Correct answer—D

Temporary memory loss and confusion are the most common side effects of ECT treatment and occur in all age-groups. Many patients experience some degree of headache, but dizziness is not a common complaint. Diarrhea and urinary incontinence generally do not occur. Some patients become nauseated and may require an antiemetic medication, but this side effect is rarely seen.

## 16 Correct answer—C

A soft, kind, but firm approach is least likely to provoke or anger the patient. Confronting the patient about her behavior is not recommended because, at this point, she cannot control her actions. Because the patient is in an agitated state, she is unable to listen or gain insight into her situation; trying to teach her about managing her money or her life is frustrating for both the nurse and the patient. Similarly, focusing on the controlled environment is ineffective while the patient remains agitated; however, this should be carried out later when the patient is less stressed.

## 17 Correct answer—B

Maintaining the patient's weight at a stable level is an appropriate initial goal while the patient is acutely manic. Once the patient is less hyperactive, the goal can be changed to reflect a gradual weight gain. Goals that use such terms as *adequate diet* or *adequate hydration* are too vaguely stated to be evaluated.

## 18 Correct answer—A

Providing easily managed food and drink for the patient to consume as she moves about her room promotes nutrition while demonstrating acceptance of the patient's inability to cease activities long enough to eat in a conventional manner. Eating in the dining room would be too stimulating at this time and might escalate the patient's behavior as well as disturb others. The nurse should not allow the patient to make her own decisions about eating but should encourage her to eat at mealtimes; patients experiencing mania tend to be too "busy" to stop for meals. Because the patient would probably view tube feedings as assaultive, they should be avoided unless no alternative is available.

## 19 Correct answer—B

While receiving lithium, the patient should maintain a regular diet with adequate fluid intake (about 70 to 100 oz [2 to 3 liters] per day). Lithium is a salt, and its retention in the body is directly influenced by the body's sodium and fluid balance. Sodium depletion must be avoided because lithium will replace sodium in the cells, leading to lithium toxicity. Low-sodium diets and high- and low-calorie diets do not provide adequate balance for proper lithium regulation.

## 20 Correct answer—B

The nurse should recognize that the patient is in the depressive phase of bipolar depression (manic-depressive disorder) and needs protection from herself because she is at risk for suicide. The nurse must always be alert for signs of self-destructive behavior and should inform the treatment team immediately so that protective measures, such as suicide precautions, can be instituted if necessary. Expressing relief at the patient's developed insight into her behavior and reportng to staff members that the she is developing insight are serious misinterpretations that miss the underlying message. Although the nurse should help C. to recognize that her behavior is a function of her bipolar disorder and not a reflection of her as a person, telling her that she has done nothing she should regret is inappropriate because it devalues her feelings.

## 21 Correct answer—D

Drawing or painting in a quiet environment provides the patient with an outlet for excess energy and encourages sublimation of feelings (transferring unacceptable aggressive drives into a constructive activity). Badminton would only increase C.'s agitation and aggression because of its competitive nature. During acute mania, the patient would be overstimulated by the noise and activity of a bingo game. Because the patient finds sitting still and concentrating difficult, working on an intricate puzzle would be too frustrating and would increase her already low self-esteem.

## 22 Correct answer—D

The serum lithium level should be maintained between 1 and 1.5 mEq/liter during the acute manic phase; therefore, the nurse should continue administering the medication. In the absence of other signs of lithium toxicity, the nurse has no need to call the physician, withhold the medication, or repeat the blood work. Nevertheless, she should continue to monitor the patient's lithium level and watch for signs of toxicity if the level begins to rise.

## 23 Correct answer—A

The nurse must remain alert for early signs of lithium toxicity, including fine tremors, nausea, vomiting, and diarrhea. When such symptoms are observed, the lithium should be withheld and the blood work repeated until the toxicity is reversed. Ataxia, confusion, and seizures indicate severe toxicity and require prompt medical management. An elevated white blood count, orthostatic hypotension, and extrapyramidal symptoms (involuntary muscle movements, restlessness, and shuffling gait) are side effects of phenothiazines, not lithium.

## 24 Correct answer—D

Mania is a mood of extreme euphoria. Delirium, the most severe state of mania, is manifested by extreme excitement, disorientation, incoherence, agitation, frantic activity, and grandiose delusions. At this stage, exhaustion, injury, and death are possible. Mild elation and hypomania are synonymous terms that refer to a lesser state of hyperactivity. Acute elation, found in severe states of mania, is evidenced by feelings of exaltation, lability, flight of ideas, talkativeness, gradiosity, inappropriate dress and makeup, urgent activity, decreased appetite and sleep, and distractibility.

## 25 Correct answer—C

M. is at increased risk for injury because of his severe hyperactivity, disorientation, and agitation. Although the nursing diagnostic categories of *Ineffective individual coping, Hopelessness,* and *Personal identity disturbance* are also appropriate, the patient's safety needs are the highest priority at this time. The nurse should take immediate action to protect the patient from injury.

## 26 Correct answer—A

Assigning M. to a room that is removed from the nurse's station helps to decrease environmental stimuli, thereby helping to reduce his level of hyperactivity. Although M.'s excessive activity may bother the nurses and other patients, the primary reason for this room assignment is to benefit M., not the others on the unit. Because a patient in any stage of mania has little or no capacity for introspection, a private room is not used for this purpose.

## 27 Correct answer—B

The patient in this situation is at increased risk for injuring herself or others. Administering a sedative as an initial intervention helps protect both the patient and the nurse from injury. Decreasing environmental stimuli is an additional measure that, when combined with medicating the patient, can reduce dangerous hyperactivity. Providing for the patient's hygiene and grooming needs is an appropriate nursing intervention, but it is not the initial priority. The overall goal is to reduce hyperactivity, so involvement in unit activities is contraindicated.

## 28 Correct answer—A

Lithium carbonate does not bind with plasma protein and is excreted exclusively through the kidneys; therefore, it is contraindicated in patients with renal system dysfunction. Lithium also is contraindicated in pregnant women and nursing mothers but not in those with reproductive disorders. Lithium can be used with caution in patients with thyroid or respiratory disorders.

## 29 Correct answer—B

An effective serum lithium level is not achieved for 7 to 10 days. Administering chlorpromazine (Thorazine) concomitantly helps control the manic symptoms during this time. Once a therapeutic lithium blood level is achieved, the chlorpromazine dosage can be reduced and discontinued. Chlorpromazine has no effect on lithium dosage. Because lithium and chlorpromazine do not have an additive effect, their efficacy is not increased when combined. Lithium toxicity is related to the body's sodium-fluid balance and would not be affected by administration of chlorpromazine.

## 30 Correct answer—B

Once the intensity of the mania has diminished, the nurse can use therapeutic confrontation in response to the patient's denial of her illness. The nurse should approach the patient on a one-to-one basis and say something like, "I overheard you say your were a journalist posing as a patient. Why don't we sit and talk about the reasons for your admission and how you are doing now." While confronting but not arguing with K., the nurse can review the reasons she was admitted and present the reality of the situation. This is more therapeutic than ignoring the comment, isolating the patient, or supporting her denial.

# CHAPTER 5

# Psychotic Disorders

# Questions

**1** Which medication is most likely to be prescribed for an outpatient with a diagnosis of chronic undifferentiated schizophrenia and a history of medication noncompliance?

A. Chlorpromazine (Thorazine)
B. Imipramine (Tofranil)
C. Lithium carbonate (Lithane)
D. Fluphenazine decanoate (Prolixin Decanoate)

**2** A patient's medication order reads: "Thioridazine (Mellaril) 200 mg orally four times a day and 100 mg orally as needed." Based on this order, the nurse should:

A. Administer the medication as prescribed
B. Question the physician about the order
C. Administer the order for 200 mg orally four times a day but not for 100 mg orally as needed
D. Administer the medication as prescribed but closely observe the patient for adverse effects

**3** The extrapyramidal effects associated with antipsychotic agents can be controlled by which medication?

A. Perphenazine (Trilafon)
B. Doxepin (Sinequan)
C. Amantadine (Symmetrel)
D. Clorazepate dipotassium (Tranxene)

**4** Which non-antipsychotic medication is used to treat some patients with schizoaffective disorder?

A. Phenelzine sulfate (Nardil)
B. Chlordiazepoxide (Librium)
C. Lithium carbonate
D. Imipramine

---

## SITUATION

*T.S., a 19-year-old sophomore, walks into the college health center and asks to speak with a counselor or therapist. For the past month, she has been having difficulty concentrating, and her grades have declined because of this. She finds herself daydream-*

*ing, lost in her own thoughts, and feeling out of it both in class
and out.*

*Questions 5 to 12 refer to this situation.*

**5** The nurse prepares to conduct the patient interview and initial
evaluation. How should she begin?

**A.** "Hello, T., I'm R.N., a nurse here at the health center. I need to
learn more about you and your reasons for coming in. Then we'll
discuss how the health center can help you"
**B.** "Hi, T. My name is R. Why don't we sit and chat for awhile.
How can I help you?"
**C.** "Ms. S., I'm the nurse assigned to interview you. If necessary,
the psychiatrist also will evaluate you today. Otherwise, you'll
see him another time"
**D.** "Ms. S., I'm Mrs. N., a nurse. You mentioned that you feel out
of it. Can you tell me more about this?"

**6** T. begins to tell the nurse about herself. Which statement indicates
possible difficulties in relating to others?

**A.** "I miss my parents and friends at home very much and feel
homesick"
**B.** "I have only two close friends at college and consider myself a
shy person"
**C.** "My roommate at college is all right, but I don't consider her a
real friend"
**D.** "I consider myself a loner and prefer reading and studying to
going out and socializing"

**7** In recounting her family history, T. suddenly begins crying and
says, "My mother was schizophrenic. She was in and out of the
hospital for years. That's not what's wrong with me, is it?" The
nurse should respond by saying:

**A.** "What makes you think you're schizophrenic like your
mother?"
**B.** "It's really too soon to tell, but heredity may play a role in
schizophrenia"
**C.** "Schizophrenia is a chronic illness, and since this is the first
time you're having a problem, I doubt if you're schizophrenic"
**D.** "I'm not yet sure what your problem is"

**8** When T. returns to the health center 1 week later, she tells the nurse that she is not sure whether anything can be done to help her. How should the nurse respond?

**A.** "You certainly are down in the dumps. You must have had a lousy week"
**B.** "I wish you would give us a chance. We really do have an excellent staff here"
**C.** "Let's talk about the reasons you seem to be feeling so hopeless right now"
**D.** "That is a very self-defeating attitude. You can't be helped unless you want to be"

**9** T. tells the nurse that she feels she cannot handle her schoolwork. Her grades have gone from A's and B's to C's, and she even may be failing a course. T. asks the nurse if she should withdraw from all her classes. Which response is most helpful?

**A.** "Do you really think withdrawing from all your classes would be best right now?"
**B.** "We can discuss the choices you have and the pros and cons of each"
**C.** "I think you should discuss this with your professors before making such a decision"
**D.** "If you are feeling so overwhelmed by the demands of your classes, that might be the best thing to do"

**10** During one of her sessions with the nurse, T. mentions that her roommate borrowed her favorite dress without asking and then ruined it by spilling grease on it. She describes this episode in a matter-of-fact way and denies feeling angry about the incident. Then she adds, "I rarely get angry at anyone." To explore the patient's feelings, the nurse should say:

**A.** "You are a very nice person not to feel angry about having your best dress ruined like that"
**B.** "I can't believe you aren't angry or at least annoyed by your roommate's behavior. Why don't you level with me?"
**C.** "I think I'd be angry about something like that. What were your thoughts when you first found out about it?"
**D.** "You know anger is a normal response to events like that. Tell me how you really feel about what she did"

**11** T. eventually is able to admit that she was somewhat annoyed by her roommate's actions and recognizes that she feels uncomfortable getting angry even when she probably should. Which initial patient goal is most appropriate?

**A.** The patient will express her anger to her roommate regarding the ruined dress
**B.** The patient will be able to ask her roommate to replace the damaged dress
**C.** The patient will begin to identify and discuss with the nurse events that arouse her feelings of anger
**D.** The patient will demonstrate that she has learned to repress her angry feelings

**12** T. continues her weekly sessions at the health center. She does not exhibit any psychotic symptoms, and her primary difficulties involve establishing and maintaining relationships with others and denying her anger. A medical diagnosis of personality disorder is considered. Based on the above symptoms and her knowledge of the disorder, the nurse would suspect the patient to have which type of personality disorder?

**A.** Schizoid
**B.** Schizotypal
**C.** Borderline
**D.** Antisocial

---

## SITUATION

*J., a 32-year-old man with a 5-year history of multiple psychiatric admissions, is brought to the emergency department by the police. He was found wandering the streets, disheveled, shoeless, and confused. Based on his previous medical records and current behavior, he is diagnosed as having chronic undifferentiated schizophrenia.*

*Questions 13 to 23 refer to this situation.*

**13** J. is escorted to the psychiatric unit by an aide. The nurse observes him sitting in the hall looking frightened. He is curled up in a corner of the bench with his arms over his head and covering his face. How should the nurse approach the patient?

**A.** Walk over to the bench, sit beside him quietly, and place an arm around his shoulders; then say, "I'm the nurse," and wait for a response
**B.** Allow him to remain alone on the bench, where he can observe the unit for a half hour or so until he is more comfortable
**C.** Greet him warmly saying, "Hi. I'm the nurse. This is a very nice unit. I think you'll like it here. Let me show you around"
**D.** Sit about 3 or 4 feet from him on the bench and say, "Hello, J. I'm a nurse on this unit. You appear frightened"; then wait for a response

**14** J. responds to the nurse by curling up on the bench even tighter. His arms still cover his head, and his hands are clasped tightly over his ears. The nurse should:

**A.** Show acceptance of J.'s behavior by remaining with him and reassuring him, gently stroking his arms and shoulders
**B.** Tell J. that she will leave him for a while and will return later when he feels more relaxed
**C.** Say gently, "J., I'll just sit here quietly with you for a while," then remain seated nearby
**D.** Say "J., most people feel uncomfortable in hospitals. You shouldn't be afraid. I'm here to help you"

**15** Later that evening, the nurse finds J. crouched in the corner of his room, with a curtain covering him. His roommate is sitting on the bed laughing and saying, "This guy is really a nut. He should be in a padded cell." How should the nurse respond to the roommate?

**A.** Say, "I'm sure J.'s behavior is frightening to you. I understand that you are trying to cover up how you really feel by laughing"
**B.** Say, "I'd appreciate it if you'd step outside for awhile. I'd like to talk with you after I help J."
**C.** Say nothing and attend to J.
**D.** Say, in a neutral tone, "I think your laughing is making J. feel worse. How would you feel if you were J.?"

**16** What is the least threatening approach to J. while he sits huddled under the curtain?

**A.** Sit next to him on the floor without speaking, and wait for him to acknowledge the nurse
**B.** Gently remove the curtain and say, "J., this is the nurse. What happened?"
**C.** Approach J. slowly and say, "J., this is the nurse. You appear to be very frightened. Can you tell me what you are experiencing?"
**D.** Call for assistance and do not approach J. until at least two other staff members are present

**17** Which is the priority nursing diagnostic category based on J.'s current behavior?

**A.** Anxiety
**B.** Impaired verbal communication
**C.** Altered thought processes
**D.** Dressing and grooming self-care deficit

**18** Because J. has previously responded well to treatment with haloperidol (Haldol), the physician orders haloperidol 10 mg orally twice a day. Which adverse effect is most common with this medication?

**A.** Extrapyramidal symptoms
**B.** Hypotension
**C.** Drowsiness
**D.** Tardive dyskinesia

**19** During the next several days, J. is observed laughing, yelling, and talking to himself. His behavior is characteristic of:

**A.** Delusion
**B.** Looseness of association
**C.** Illusion
**D.** Hallucination

**20** J. tells the nurse, "The earth is doomed, you know. The ozone layer is being destroyed by hair spray. You should get away before you die." J. appears frightened as he says this. The most helpful response is to:

A. Say, "J., I think you are overreacting. I know there is some concern about the earth's ozone layer, but there is no immediate danger to anyone"
B. Say, "I've heard about the destruction of the ozone layer and its effect on the earth. Why don't you tell me more about it?"
C. Ignore J.'s statement and redirect his attention to some activity on the unit
D. Say, "J., are you saying you feel as though something bad will happen to you?"

**21** After a half hour, J. continues to ramble about the ozone layer and being doomed to die. He paces in an increasingly agitated manner, and he begins to speak more loudly. At this time, the nurse should:

A. Check to see whether the physician ordered haloperidol on an as-needed basis
B. Allow J. to continue pacing but observe him closely
C. Try to involve J. in a current events discussion group that is about to start
D. Tell J. to go to his room for a while

**22** The treatment team reviews J.'s behavior and decides to continue increasing his haloperidol dosage for the next few weeks. The nurse must closely observe the patient for:

A. Signs of haloperidol toxicity
B. Evidence of the therapeutic window effect
C. Increased incidence of orthostatic hypotension
D. Indications of tardive dyskinesia

**23** After several months, J. improves, and the physician decides to change the medication to haloperidol decanoate (Haldol Decanoate). Why is this change made?

A. Haloperidol decanoate is more effective
B. Haloperidol decanoate has fewer side effects
C. A change in medication produces a better response
D. Haloperidol decanoate can be given monthly instead of daily

---

**SITUATION**

*L., a 28-year-old woman, has been hospitalized for most of the past 12 years. For the past 2¹/₂ years, she has been on a unit for chronically mentally ill patients. Her psychiatric diagnosis is disorganized type schizophrenia. Her behavior is labile, fluctuating from childishness to incoherence to loud yelling to making growling noises to demonstrating slow but appropriate interaction. L. needs assistance with all her activities of daily living (ADLs). In the morning, she remains in her nightgown unless helped to dress.*

*Questions 24 to 26 refer to this situation.*

**24** Which behavior is characteristic of a patient with disorganized type schizophrenia?

**A.** Extreme social impairment
**B.** Suspicious delusions
**C.** Waxy flexibility
**D.** Appropriate affect

**25** L. continues to be unable to complete her ADLs without staff direction and assistance. The nurse formulates a nursing diagnosis of *Dressing and grooming self-care deficit related to inability to function without assistance.* An appropriate patient goal is that within 1 month, L. will be able to:

**A.** Complete ADLs independently
**B.** Complete ADLs with only verbal encouragement
**C.** Complete ADLs with assistance in organizing her grooming items and clothing
**D.** Complete ADLs with complete assistance

**26** L. is seen sitting in the day room looking disheveled. Her slacks are stained and her blouse is incorrectly buttoned so that one side hangs several inches below the other. The nurse can help L. most by:

**A.** Telling her that her slacks are soiled and her blouse needs to be rebuttoned
**B.** Taking her to her room, selecting another pair of slacks, and fixing her blouse
**C.** Reminding her that she should complete her ADLs before going to the dayroom
**D.** Bringing her to a mirror and helping her identify what needs to be corrected

## SITUATION

*M., a 24-year-old college student, is brought to the hospital by her boyfriend with whom she has been living for the past 6 months. He reports that M.'s behavior has become very strange over the past week. She has become more and more withdrawn to the point that yesterday she sat on a chair in her room with her eyes closed, not moving for 6 hours, until he carried her to bed. He says that at first he thought she was just depressed about the recent death of a friend, but now he thinks she's "flipped out." M. is admitted with a diagnosis of catatonic schizophrenia.*

*Questions 27 to 32 refer to this situation.*

**27** During the physical assessment, M.'s arm remains outstretched after her pulse and blood pressure are taken, and the nurse must reposition it for her. The patient is manifesting:

**A.** Suggestibility
**B.** Negativity
**C.** Waxy flexibility
**D.** Retardation

**28** M. keeps her eyes closed and does not respond to questions from the nurse or the physician. The nurse must keep in mind that:

**A.** The patient is aware of what is going on around her and could respond if she wanted
**B.** The patient may be able to hear what is happening around her even though she does not respond
**C.** The patient cannot hear or comprehend what is being said to her
**D.** The patient is in a regressed state and should be treated like a frightened child

**29** M. remains in bed with her eyes closed. She continues to be unresponsive and does not eat or drink. The physician orders chlorpromazine (Thorazine) 100 mg orally four times a day. Under these circumstances, the nurse should:

**A.** Withhold the medication until the patient becomes more responsive and eats
**B.** Administer the appropriate dose of chlorpromazine in a concentrate form
**C.** Administer the chlorpromazine as needed
**D.** Request an order for chlorpromazine to be administered intramuscularly

**30** While M. remains in an unresponsive state, the nurse's highest priority is to assess the patient's:

**A.** Fluid intake and output
**B.** Daily activity level
**C.** Communication level
**D.** Response to others

**31** One evening, M. suddenly begins running up and down the hall. She strips off her clothing and strikes out wildly at anyone she passes. This incident of catatonic excitement is considered:

**A.** A response to increased activity on the unit
**B.** A self-limiting episode that will subside as suddenly as it began
**C.** An occurrence related to internal not external stimuli
**D.** An indication of patient improvement

**32** All of the following interventions would be appropriate for a patient experiencing catatonic excitement *except:*

**A.** Clearing the area of other patients
**B.** Calling for the assistance of at least three other staff members
**C.** Obtaining an order for and preparing an as-needed dose of chlorpromazine
**D.** Restraining the patient and calling for help

## SITUATION

*H., age 40, is brought to the hospital by his wife, who states that for the past week her husband has refused all meals and accused her of trying to poison him. She claims that before this drastic*

*change in behavior, he became withdrawn, forgetful, and inatten-*
*tive and had frequent mood swings. During the initial interview,*
*H. appears suspicious. His speech, which is only partly compre-*
*hensible, reveals that his thoughts are controlled by delusions of*
*possession by the devil. He claims that the devil told him that peo-*
*ple around him are trying to destroy him and that he should trust*
*no one. The physician diagnoses paranoid schizophrenia and ad-*
*mits the patient to the psychiatric unit.*

*Questions 33 to 43 refer to this situation.*

**33** Schizophrenia is best described as a disorder characterized by:

**A.** Disturbed relationships related to an inability to communicate and think clearly
**B.** Severe mood swings and periods of low to high activity
**C.** Multiple personalities, one of which is more destructive than the others
**D.** Auditory and visual hallucinations

**34** The nursing assessment of H. should include careful observation of his:

**A.** Thinking, perceiving, and decision-making skills
**B.** Verbal and nonverbal communication processes
**C.** Affect and behavior
**D.** Psychomotor activity

**35** The patient's thought content can be evaluated on the basis of which assessment area?

**A.** Presence or absence of delusions
**B.** Unbiased information from the patient's psychiatric history
**C.** Degree of orientation to person, place, and time
**D.** Ability to think abstractly

**36** Nursing care for a psychotic patient must be based on valid psychiatric and nursing theories. The nurse's interpersonal communication with the patient and specific nursing interventions must be:

**A.** Flexible enough for the nurse to adjust the nursing care plan as the situation warrants
**B.** Clearly identified, with boundaries and specifically defined roles
**C.** Warm and nonthreatening
**D.** Centered on clearly defined limits and expression of empathy

**37** After 2 days on the unit, H. continues to refuse to eat any hospital meals. He has been observed drinking soda and juices bought from a vending machine in the hospital lobby. Which approach is best at this time?

**A.** Have staff members eat meals with H., encouraging him to eat and demonstrating that the food is not poisoned
**B.** Set firm limits with H., restricting his access to vending machine items until he begins to eat at least part of his meals
**C.** Express concern to H. about his refusal to eat but allow him to control what and when he eats while continuing to observe and monitor him
**D.** Ignore H.'s refusal to eat and recognize that he will eat when he is hungry

**38** Although H. refuses to eat, he continues to take his medication. Considering his suspicious behavior and delusions, what is the best way to administer his medication?

**A.** Administer all medications parenterally to ensure adequate dosage
**B.** Administer medication only in liquid form to eliminate the possibility of the patient not swallowing his tablets
**C.** Administer a combination of liquid and tablets to ensure that the patient is getting at least some medication
**D.** Administer the medication in the same form each time

**39** The nurse observes H. pacing in his room. He is alone but talking in an angry tone. When asked what he was experiencing, he replies, "The devil is yelling in my ear. He says people here want to hurt me." The nurse's best response is:

**A.** "Can you tell me more about what the devil is saying to you?"
**B.** "How do you feel when the devil says such things to you?"
**C.** "I don't hear any voice, H. Are you feeling afraid right now?"
**D.** "H., the devil cannot talk to you"

**40** H. has been hearing voices for many years. An approach that has proven effective is for the hallucinating patient to:

**A.** Practice saying "Go away" or "Stop" when he hears voices
**B.** Take an as-needed dose of his psychotropic medication whenever he hears voices
**C.** Sing loudly to drown out the voices and to distract himself
**D.** Go to his room until the voices go away

**41** H. requests that his room be changed. He states that his roommate is homosexual and has been making advances to him. He wants to be in a private room. How should the nurse reply?

**A.** Remind H. that he is in a hospital and not a hotel and tell him that patients are assigned to rooms on the basis of need
**B.** Tell H. that his request will be discussed that morning and if a room is available he will be moved
**C.** Inform H. that his roommate is not homosexual and that he should get to know him better
**D.** Ask H. if he is physically attracted to his roommate

**42** Physical activity is an important part of the schizophrenic patient's treatment plan. Assuming H. is capable of the following activities, which one is most appropriate for him?

**A.** Taking a daily brisk walk with a staff member
**B.** Playing a basketball game
**C.** Participating in touch football
**D.** Shooting basketballs with another patient and a staff member

**43** Plans are being made for H.'s discharge. His wife expresses concern over whether her husband will continue to take his prescribed medication. The nurse should inform her that:

**A.** Her concern is valid but H. is an adult and has the right to make his own decisions
**B.** She can easily mix the medication in H.'s food if he stops taking it
**C.** H. can be given a long-acting medication that is administered every 1 to 4 weeks
**D.** H. knows that he must take his medication as prescribed to avoid future hospitalizations

# Answer sheet

| | A B C D | | A B C D |
|---|---|---|---|
| 1 | ○○○○ | 31 | ○○○○ |
| 2 | ○○○○ | 32 | ○○○○ |
| 3 | ○○○○ | 33 | ○○○○ |
| 4 | ○○○○ | 34 | ○○○○ |
| 5 | ○○○○ | 35 | ○○○○ |
| 6 | ○○○○ | 36 | ○○○○ |
| 7 | ○○○○ | 37 | ○○○○ |
| 8 | ○○○○ | 38 | ○○○○ |
| 9 | ○○○○ | 39 | ○○○○ |
| 10 | ○○○○ | 40 | ○○○○ |
| 11 | ○○○○ | 41 | ○○○○ |
| 12 | ○○○○ | 42 | ○○○○ |
| 13 | ○○○○ | 43 | ○○○○ |
| 14 | ○○○○ | | |
| 15 | ○○○○ | | |
| 16 | ○○○○ | | |
| 17 | ○○○○ | | |
| 18 | ○○○○ | | |
| 19 | ○○○○ | | |
| 20 | ○○○○ | | |
| 21 | ○○○○ | | |
| 22 | ○○○○ | | |
| 23 | ○○○○ | | |
| 24 | ○○○○ | | |
| 25 | ○○○○ | | |
| 26 | ○○○○ | | |
| 27 | ○○○○ | | |
| 28 | ○○○○ | | |
| 29 | ○○○○ | | |
| 30 | ○○○○ | | |

## Answers and rationales

**1** Correct answer—**D**

Fluphenazine decanoate (Prolixin Decanoate) is a long-acting anti-psychotic agent given by injection. Because it has a 4-week duration of action, fluphenazine is commonly prescribed for outpatients with a history of medication noncompliance. The antipsychotic agent chlorpromazine (Thorazine) must be administered daily to maintain adequate plasma levels, which necessitates compliance with the dosage schedule. Imipramine (Tofranil), a tricyclic antidepressant, and lithium carbonate (Lithane), a mood stabilizer, are generally not used to treat patients with chronic schizophrenia.

**2** Correct answer—**B**

The nurse must question this order immediately. Thioridazine (Mellaril) has an absolute dosage ceiling of 800 mg/day. Any dosage above this level places the patient at high risk for toxic pigmentary retinopathy, which cannot be reversed. The order, as written, allows for administering more than the maximum 800 mg/day; it should be corrected immediately, before the patient's health is jeopardized.

**3** Correct answer—**C**

Amantadine (Symmetrel) is an anticholinergic drug used to relieve drug-induced extrapyramidal adverse effects, such as muscle weakness, involuntary muscle movement, pseudoparkinsonism, and tardive dyskinesia. Other anticholinergic agents used for extrapyramidal reactions include benzotropine mesylate (Cogentin), trihexyphenidyl (Artane), biperiden (Akineton), and diphenhydramine (Benadryl). Perphenazine is an antipsychotic; doxepin, an antidepressant; and chlorazepate, an antianxiety agent. Because these medications have no anticholinergic or neurotransmitter effects, they do not alleviate extrapyramidal reactions.

**4** Correct answer—**C**

Lithium carbonate, an antimania drug, is used to treat patients with cyclical schizoaffective disorder (a psychotic disorder once classified under schizophrenia that produces affective symptoms, including maniclike activity). Lithium helps control the affective component of this disorder. Phenelzine sulfate (Nardil) is a monoamine oxidase inhibitor prescribed for patients who have not re-

sponded to other antidepressant drugs, such as imipramine. Chlordiazepoxide (Librium), an antianxiety agent, is generally contraindicated in psychotic patients. Imipramine, primarily classified as
an antidepressant agent, also is used to treat patients with agora-
phobia and those undergoing cocaine detoxification.

## 5 Correct answer—A

Each interview should begin with a clear statement of introduction
that defines the purpose of the interview. Because the patient has
come to the health center for the first time, informality, use of first
names only, and an invitation to sit and chat are inappropriate.
Also inappropriate are introductions with last names only, using
clinical terminology, and abruptly mentioning the psychiatrist; this
type of introduction is cold and distancing. Only after the nurse
has introduced herself, defined her role, and told the patient what
to expect from the interview should she begin exploring the
patient's problem.

## 6 Correct answer—D

The patient's self-description as a loner who prefers solitary activities, such as reading and studying, over socializing clearly suggests that she may be having difficulty relating to others. Shy persons who have established and maintained relationships may
desire additional social skills but usually can relate meaningfully
to others. Feeling homesick and missing family and friends is not
unusual or abnormal; neither is not liking everyone.

## 7 Correct answer—A

The nurse should explore the basis for T.'s fear that she may be
schizophrenic because her response can provide clues to her current difficulties and self-concept. Once the nurse understands the
patient's thoughts and feelings, she can better respond to her question. Although it is true that a diagnosis cannot yet be made and
that heredity may be a factor in schizophrenia, giving the patient
this information would probably not be helpful and does not encourage the patient to express her concerns. Although schizophrenia is a chronic illness, the patient is in a vulnerable age-group
(ages 15 to 35) for the onset of the disease. The nurse should not
consider the patient schizophrenic until more data are obtained
and the physician makes a positive diagnosis.

**8** Correct answer—**C**

By reflecting T.'s apparent hopelessness and inviting her to discuss her feelings, the nurse provides an opportunity for the patient to explore her perception of the situation. Acknowledging that T. is down in the dumps and attributing this to a lousy week tells rather than asks the patient how she feels. Lecturing T. about how good the staff are or how her negative attitude will impede her progress denies her feelings and is judgmental and nontherapeutic.

**9** Correct answer—**B**

The nurse's role is to assist the patient in exploring and evaluating alternatives—not to tell the patient what she thinks is best. Encouraging her to discuss the alternatives and helping her evaluate them promotes the patient's growth. Judgmental responses, such as "Do you really think..." or "I think you should..." belittle the patient by implying that the nurse knows best. These responses also fail to encourage the patient to explore all the possible choices. The nurse should not agree with the patient's decision until the situation has been discussed and understood.

**10** Correct answer—**C**

Using self-disclosure in response to T.'s situation shows that the nurse empathizes with the patient and relays that the negative feelings are acceptable. By encouraging the patient to discuss her thoughts, the nurse seeks to release T.'s underlying feelings. Promoting T.'s denial of anger by telling her that she must be a nice person is not helpful. Confrontational approaches, such as "Level with me" and "Tell me how you really feel," would put T. on the defensive and inhibit her expression of feelings.

**11** Correct answer—**C**

T. needs to learn that it is acceptable to express her anger before she learns to talk about her feelings. The nurse is a safe, supportive person with whom T. can begin this process. Once the patient can admit her feelings to herself, she can begin expressing them more directly to others. Repression (barring of unacceptable thoughts or painful experiences from consciousness) is not a desirable goal because the patient would expend much energy containing such thoughts and have difficulty focusing on day-to-day issues.

## 12 Correct answer—A

Schizoid personality disorder is characterized by difficulty in forming social relationships and in expressing anger, preference for solitary activities, emotional detachment, daydreaming, and indecisiveness. Schizotypal personality is manifested by oddities of thinking, perception, speech, and behavior that are not severe enough to be labeled schizophrenia. Borderline personality, marked by instability in several areas of development, is evidenced by unstable mood, poor relationships, impulsivity, and self-destructive behavior. The diagnosis of antisocial personality disorder is applied only to patients older than age 18 who have a history of conduct disorder before age 18. Conduct disorders are characterized by behaviors such as truancy, lying, problems in school, and running away.

## 13 Correct answer—D

In approaching J. for the first time, the nurse should keep in mind that schizophrenic patients fear closeness. Moving too close to the patient at first may be seen as an invasion of his personal space, which could frighten him and cause him to strike out at the nurse. To avoid overwhelming J., the nurse should limit her introduction to who she is and acknowledge that the patient appears frightened. Touch can have unpredictable meanings to a frightened psychiatric patient, so it is best to avoid it, especially with someone new. Because J. is obviously in distress, the nurse should gently intervene rather than leave him alone or ignore his distress with false reassurance about how nice the unit is.

## 14 Correct answer—C

The nurse should attempt to establish trust by demonstrating acceptance of J.'s behavior and offering to remain with him. This lets J. know that he does not have to talk to get her attention. Touching or stroking the patient ignores the indications that he is trying to distance himself as a protective measure and would be viewed as intrusive and threatening. Because the patient's behavior results from his resistance to closeness, leaving him alone would reinforce this conduct and would add to his anxiety. Attempts to offer verbal reassurance are likely to be ineffective for a withdrawn and frightened patient such as J.

## 15 Correct answer—B

Because the nurse's first priority is to attend to J., the most appropriate action is to ask the roommate to step outside. The nurse should recognize the roommate's behavior as a probable sign of increased anxiety and should ask the roommate to leave without engaging him in a prolonged discussion. However, she should confront the roommate as soon as possible to discuss his reaction to J.'s behavior and to explore more appropriate responses. Any attempt to interpret the roommate's behavior at this time could escalate his anxiety about the situation and cause additional outbursts that could further increase J.'s anxiety.

## 16 Correct answer—C

J.'s behavior indicates that he is experiencing severe anxiety and panic. The nurse can avoid startling him by approaching him slowly while talking to him, yet maintaining a safe distance of 3' to 4' (about 1 to 1.5 m). Although sitting at the same level as the patient can facilitate communication, failing to maintain a safe distance may place the nurse at considerable risk should the patient suddenly become violent. The nurse should encourage J. to discuss his present experience by reflecting her observations of his behavior. She should not attempt to remove the curtain, which is being used to protect against intrusion. As J.'s anxiety decreases, he can be asked to remove it himself. Additional staff members should be called if the patient does not tolerate the nurse's approach and becomes agitated; however, initially, their presence would probably frighten him more.

## 17 Correct answer—A

The priority nursing diagnostic category is *Anxiety,* severe to panic-level, as evidenced by J.'s extreme withdrawal and attempt to protect himself from the environment. The nurse must act immediately to reduce his anxiety and to protect the patient and others from possible injury. *Impaired verbal communication,* as evidenced by noncommunicativeness, *Altered thought processes,* as evidenced by an inability to understand the situation, and *Dressing and grooming self-care deficit,* as evidenced by a disheveled appearance, are all appropriate nursing diagnostic categories but are not the priority in this situation.

## 18 Correct answer—A

Extrapyramidal effects, including dystonia, akathisia, pseudoparkinsonism, and tremors, are the most common adverse reactions associated with haloperidol (Haldol), a high-potency antipsychotic drug. Haloperidol rarely causes tardive dyskinesia, a severe, irreversible extrapyramidal reaction. Hypotension and drowsiness are common side effects of low-potency antipsychotic agents, such as chlorpromazine and thioridazine.

## 19 Correct answer—D

Auditory hallucination, hearing voices when there are no external stimuli, is common in schizophrenic patients. The nurse can indirectly determine that J. is hallucinating by observing such behaviors as laughing, yelling, and talking to himself. Delusions, false beliefs or ideas that arise without external stimuli, also are common in patients with schizophrenia. For example, a delusional patient may believe that he is being controlled by the television in his room. Schizophrenic patients may exhibit looseness of association, a pattern of thinking and communicating in which ideas are not clearly linked to one another. For example, the patient may make statements that are disconnected and unclear to the listener. A less severe perceptual disturbance is illusion, wherein the patient misinterprets actual external stimuli. For example, the patient may see a red exit sign and think that the wall is on fire. Illusions are not commonly associated with schizophrenia.

## 20 Correct answer—D

J.'s statement combines truth (the ozone layer is being destroyed), some exaggeration that may be delusional (the earth is doomed), and some projection of his own fears (the nurse should get away). By choosing to respond to the underlying message about J.'s fear of being destroyed, the nurse attempts to help him identify and express his feelings in a more direct and appropriate manner. Reflecting doubt about delusional statements can help the patient see that the nurse does not share his belief. However, such reflection should not be stated judgmentally ("You are overreacting") or in a way that denies his feelings ("There is no danger"). Pursuing a discussion about the ozone layer or ignoring his comments completely are nontherapeutic approaches because they do not acknowledge his fear.

## 21 Correct answer—A

Because interpersonal interventions have failed to decrease J.'s
anxiety level, medication is needed. If an as-needed order is un-
available, the nurse should ask the physician to write one. If the
nurse does not intervene and allows J. to continue pacing, his anxiety and agitation may escalate, which may be dangerous to the patient and others. Involving J. in a discussion group would probably increase his anxiety level and cause him to act out
aggressively. Telling J. to go to his room *after* he receives his medication would be helpful; the combination of an antipsychotic
agent and reduced stimuli will help to decrease his agitation.

## 22 Correct answer—B

The therapeutic window effect is the point at which an increase in
dosage decreases a drug's therapeutic effect. Therefore, the nurse
must closely observe the patient as the haloperidol dosage is increased. The toxic level of haloperidol has not been clearly established. Orthostatic hypotension is not common with this drug; tardive dyskinesia is rare. A patient receiving haloperidol is typically
observed for therapeutic effects rather than intolerable side effects.

## 23 Correct answer—D

Haloperidol decanoate (Haldol Decanoate), given by depot injection, has a 4-week duration of action, which makes it appropriate
for patients who require long-term drug therapy. Haloperidol
decanoate is not more effective; nor is it useful for treating patients with acute psychotic episodes because a therapeutic level is
not achieved for up to 3 months. Although this form of haloperidol rarely causes sedation or postural hypotension, it often produces extrapyramidal symptoms. Switching antipsychotic agents
does not achieve a better response; high-potency antipsychotic
drugs are equivalent in clinical effectiveness.

## 24 Correct answer—A

Disorganized type schizophrenia (formerly hebephrenia) is characterized by extreme social impairment, marked inappropriate affect, silliness, grimacing, posturing, and fragmented delusions and
hallucinations. A patient with a paranoid disorder typically exhibits suspicious delusions (beliefs that evil forces are after him).
Waxy flexibility, a condition in which the patient's limbs remain

fixed in uncomfortable positions for long periods, is characteristic of catatonic schizophrenia.

## 25 Correct answer—C

L.'s history of hospitalization and her disorganized personality caused by schizophrenia have affected her ability to care for herself. Interventions should be directed at helping her complete her activities of daily living (ADLs) with the assistance of staff members, who can provide needed structure by helping her select her grooming items and clothing. This goal promotes realistic independence. As L. improves and attains the established goal, new goals can be set that are directed at the patient's completing ADLs with only verbal encouragement and, ultimately, completing them independently. L.'s condition does not indicate a need for complete assistance, which would only foster dependence.

## 26 Correct answer—D

The nurse should help L. to recognize for herself what needs to be corrected. Taking her to a mirror encourages reality testing (determining objective reality) and helps develop self-perception with the nurse's support and guidance. Providing L. with an opportunity to attend to her appearance promotes mastery of ADL skills and is more therapeutic than telling her what is wrong or fixing her clothes for her.

## 27 Correct answer—C

Waxy flexibility—an ability to assume and maintain awkward or uncomfortable positions for long periods—is characteristic of catatonic schizophrenia. Patients often remain in these awkward positions until repositioned by someone else. Patients with dependency problems may demonstrate suggestibility, a response pattern in which the patient easily agrees to the ideas and suggestions of others rather than making his own independent judgments. Negativity (resistance, for example, to being moved or being asked to cooperate) and retardation (slowed movement) are also seen in catatonic patients.

## 28 Correct answer—B

The nurse should assume that a withdrawn, unresponsive patient may be able to hear what is being said and what is going on around her. She should address the patient by name, tell her what is being done, and orient her to person, place, and time. All staff members should be respectful of the patient's condition and careful when conversing in the patient's presence. The patient's withdrawal is an extreme defense mechanism that is not consciously controlled and therefore is not willful. Consistent and caring interventions can help the patient develop trust and eventually reduce the need for such extreme behavior. Although the patient may experience extreme anxiety and fear, treating her like a child is inappropriate and reinforces dependency.

## 29 Correct answer—D

Because the physician has ordered chlorpromazine (Thorazine) to be administered orally and the patient is not eating or drinking, the nurse should request an order for I.M. administration instead. Giving oral forms of medication (including tablets and concentrates) while the patient is in this state would be unsafe and would not ensure that the proper dose is being received. After administering the I.M. dose, the nurse should closely monitor the patient's vital signs; postural hypotension is a possible side effect. The patient requires adequate doses of chlorpromazine, an antipsychotic, to relieve her symptoms; giving this drug on an as-needed basis would not ensure the proper dosage necessary for a therapeutic effect.

## 30 Correct answer—A

The nurse should monitor M.'s fluid intake and output closely. The patient's refusal to eat or drink and her limited mobility put her at high risk for severe fluid and electrolyte imbalance, dehydration, inadequate nutrition, constipation, and urine retention. Vital signs and skin assessment can also indicate fluid volume deficit. Assessing the patient's activity level, communication level, and response to others is of secondary importance.

## 31 Correct answer—C

Catatonic excitement, which is characterized by extreme purposeless motor activity, agitation, and striking out wildly, appears related to internal rather than external stimuli. It differs from manic excitement, which is escalated by environmental stimuli (and therefore is somewhat more predictable) and can be lessened by a quiet setting. Catatonic excitement is not self-limiting; it may not stop without intervention. A patient experiencing catatonic excitement needs immediate attention to protect herself and others from injury; it does not indicate improvement.

## 32 Correct answer—**D**

A patient experiencing catatonic excitement is extremely agitated and potentially dangerous to herself and others. The nurse should not attempt to restrain the patient without adequate assistance. At least three staff members should approach the patient and have a plan for restraint, if needed. While waiting for staff backup, the area should be cleared of other patients as well as chairs or objects that could be thrown or pose a safety hazard. The nurse should prepare an as-needed injection of chlorpromazine, if ordered, so that the patient can be medicated once safely restrained.

## 33 Correct answer—**A**

Schizophrenia can best be described as one of a group of psychotic reactions characterized by disturbances in an individual's relationship with people and an inability to communicate and think clearly. Schizophrenic thoughts, feelings, and behavior are commonly evidenced by withdrawal, fluctuating moods, disordered thinking, and regressive tendencies. Severe mood swings and periods of low to high activity are typical of bipolar disorder. Multiple personality, which is sometimes confused with schizophrenia, is a dissociative personality disorder, not a psychotic illness. Many schizophrenic patients have auditory, not visual, hallucinations. Visual hallucinations are more common in organic or toxic disorders.

## 34 Correct answer—**A**

The nursing assessment of a psychotic patient requires careful inquiry about and observation of his thinking, perceiving, symbolizing, and decision-making skills and abilities. Assessment of such a patient typically reveals alterations in thought content and process, perception, affect, and psychomotor behavior; changes in personality, coping, and sense of self; lack of self-motivation; presence of psychosocial stressors; and degeneration of adaptive functioning. Although assessing the patient's communication processes, affect, behavior, and psychomotor activity would reveal important information about the patient's condition, the nurse should concentrate on determining whether the patient is hallucinating by assessing his thought processes and decision-making ability.

## 35 Correct answer—A

Because delusions constitute the major disturbance in thought content, the nurse should base her assessment on their presence or absence. Although patients may report delusions spontaneously, specific questioning usually is required. Clues suggesting the presence of delusions are evasiveness, suspicion, and other indications of sensitivity to interview questions. The nurse cannot effectively evaluate the patient's thought content from his history. A patient can be oriented to person, place, and time yet still have delusions. Abstract thinking, the ability to infer beyond the literal and concrete meaning of words, reflects the patient's type of thinking, not its content.

## 36 Correct answer—A

A flexible care plan is needed for any patient who behaves in a suspicious, withdrawn, or regressed way or who has a thought disorder. Because such a patient communicates at different levels and is in control of himself at various times, the nurse must be able to adjust the nursing care as the situation warrants. The nurse's role should be clear; however, the boundaries or limits of her role should be flexible enough to meet patient needs. Because a schizophrenic patient fears closeness and affection, a warm approach may be too threatening at this time. Expressing empathy is important, but centering interventions on clearly defined limits is impossible because the patient's situation can change without warning.

## 37 Correct answer—C

The nurse must avoid a power struggle with H. about his eating habits to prevent any further escalation of paranoia. The patient should be allowed to eat what he chooses as long as no coexisting medical problem, such as diabetes or a compromised fluid and electrolyte status, is present. However, the nurse should monitor the patient's physical status closely. As H. begins to trust the environment and those in it and as his psychotic symptoms subside with medication, he will begin to eat. H.'s delusions about food poisoning probably will not be corrected by having staff members eat with him or by setting firm limits. These activities may heighten his suspicion and augment his paranoid behavior. The nurse should not ignore H.'s behavior or assume that he will eat eventually; doing so could place the patient at risk for dehydration and malnutrition.

## 38 Correct answer—D

Paranoid patients are hypersensitive to changes in routines and established patterns. Consistency on the part of the nurse and other staff members fosters trust and security. Medication should be administered in the same form each time—for example, the same number of tablets with the same type of juice. Parenteral routes are generally used only when the patient refuses oral medication or is extremely agitated. Liquid psychotropic agents can be distasteful but may be ordered if the nurse suspects that the patient is not swallowing his tablets. The nurse should not give the patient a combination of liquid and tablets because it may confuse him.

## 39 Correct answer—C

When dealing with a hallucinating patient, the nurse should assess the patient's needs and reflect reality by telling him that she does not hear or share his perception. Because hallucinations are generally projections of the patient's own unconscious thoughts and feelings, the nurse should not deny the patient's experience. However, asking about the voices in a way that implies the nurse agrees with their reality is nontherapeutic. Telling H. that the devil cannot talk to him is confrontational and judgmental.

## 40 Correct answer—A

Researchers have found that most patients can learn to control bothersome hallucinations by telling the voices to go away or stop. Since H. has been hearing voices for many years, this approach would be appropriate for him. Taking an as-needed dose of psychotropic medication whenever he hears voices may lead to overmedication and put him at risk for adverse effects, such as extrapyramidal symptoms. Because it is unlikely that H. will become totally free of the voices, he must learn to deal with the hallucinations without relying on medication. Although distraction is helpful, singing loudly may upset other patients and will be socially unacceptable after the patient is discharged. Hallucinations are most bothersome when it is quiet and the patient is alone, so going to his room would increase rather than decrease the hallucinations.

## 41 Correct answer—B

Telling H. that his request for a room change will be discussed with other team members is an honest and factual response. Paranoid patients are commonly disturbed by doubts about gender identity, which is expressed as beliefs that others think they are homosexual or that others are making homosexual advances to them. A change of room would be appropriate if possible. Responding by telling the patient that he is not in a hotel would be inappropriate and only serve to alienate him from the staff. Attempting to dissuade the patient from his beliefs by telling him that his roommate is not homosexual or confronting him about his possible attraction to his roommate would further increase his anxiety.

## 42 Correct answer—A

The patient should be encouraged to participate in a noncompetitive and nonthreatening physical activity. A brisk walk with a staff member best meets H.'s activity needs at this time. Activities such as basketball and touch football should be avoided because they require the patient to have physical contact with others, particularly other men. Since H. has already expressed some homosexual concerns, these activities would be threatening to him.

## 43 Correct answer—C

Medications such as fluphenazine decanoate (Prolixin Decanoate), fluphenazine enanthate (Prolixin Enanthate), and haloperidol decanoate (Haldol Decanoate) are long-acting psychotropic drugs that are given by depot injection every 1 to 4 weeks. These agents are especially useful for noncompliant patients because they are not given daily and their effect can be monitored when the patient receives his injection at the outpatient clinic. This arrangement also puts less stress on family members by alleviating the burden of having to monitor the patient's compliance with the medication regimen. A patient has the right to refuse medication, but this issue is not the focus of discussion at this time. Medication should never be hidden in food or drink to trick the patient into taking it. Besides destroying the patient's trust, it places the patient at risk for overmedication or undermedication because the amount administered is difficult to determine. Assuming that the patient knows he must take his medication as prescribed to avoid future hospitalizations is unrealistic; many schizophrenic patients are noncompliant and require close monitoring by family members.

# CHAPTER 6

# Violent Behavior

## Questions

**1** Mental health laws in each state specify when restraints can be used and which type of restraints are allowed. Most laws stipulate that restraints can be used:

**A.** For a maximum of 2 hours
**B.** As necessary to control the patient
**C.** If the patient is a present danger to himself or others
**D.** Only with the patient's consent

**2** A patient at highest risk for suicide is one who:

**A.** Appears depressed, frequently thinks of dying, and gives away all personal possessions
**B.** Plans a violent death and has the means readily available
**C.** Tells others that he might do something if life does not get better soon
**D.** Talks about wanting to die

**3** Which group is considered at high risk for suicide?

**A.** Adolescents, men over age 45, and previous suicide attempters
**B.** Teachers, divorced persons, and substance abusers
**C.** Alcohol abusers, widows, and young married men
**D.** Depressed persons, physicians, and persons living in rural areas

**4** Which characteristic is most common among suicidal patients?

**A.** Ambivalence
**B.** Remorse
**C.** Anger
**D.** Psychosis

---

### SITUATION

*L.C., age 29, is brought to the emergency department by her husband, who found her in the bathroom slitting her wrists when he returned home from a job interview. The couple has been married for 8 years. Mr. C., a previously successful lawyer, was fired from his job 1 year ago. At that time, their marriage became tense and stressful. Mr. C. blames his wife for his job loss and for being unsupportive. Usually responsible and level-headed, L. has been de-*

*veloping low self-esteem and an inability to cope with menial
tasks, driving her to despair and feelings of impending doom.*

*Questions 5 to 10 refer to this situation.*

**5** On admission to the surgical unit for treatment of deep lacerations
to both wrists, L. tells the nurse, "Next time, I'll make sure no one
stops me from doing what I plan to do. I don't want to be responsible for anyone's failure." How should the nurse respond?

**A.** "I don't understand. Whose failure are you responsible for?"
**B.** "We are here to make sure nothing happens to you. We will
protect you from yourself"
**C.** "Don't you realize how lucky you are that your husband found
you before you did more damage?"
**D.** "What exactly do you plan to do?"

**6** The nursing staff discusses how to implement suicide precautions
while L. is on the surgical unit. The most immediate nursing intervention is to:

**A.** Obtain a physician's order for restraints to prevent further suicide attempts
**B.** Assign a nurse to remain with L. and observe her on a one-to-
one basis
**C.** Obtain a physician's order to sedate L. to reduce suicidal ideation
**D.** Discuss the need for psychiatric consultation with the physician

**7** The nurses should implement all of the following suicide precautions for L. *except:*

**A.** Restricting all visitors, phone calls, and contact with family
members and friends
**B.** Removing all potentially dangerous and sharp objects, such as
razors, glass, scissors, electrical cords, and nail files
**C.** Explaining the procedures and reasons for suicide precautions
to the patient
**D.** Explaining the procedures for suicide precautions to all persons who have contact with the patient

**8** After her wrist wounds have healed sufficiently, L. is transferred to a locked psychiatric unit. Suicide precautions on this unit are most likely to be:

**A.** Continued at the same level as those on the surgical unit
**B.** Discontinued because it is a locked unit
**C.** Changed to 15-minute checks and restriction to the unit
**D.** Modified to allow more time for privacy

**9** Mr. C. asks the nurse, "How long will this go on? Why doesn't my wife just snap out of it and pull herself together? She has always been so well organized and responsible. I depend on her." Which response by the nurse is best?

**A.** "You need to understand that your wife has been under great pressure since you lost your job"
**B.** "It's really impossible to say how long it will take before she is feeling better. Have you told her how much you miss her?"
**C.** "It seems to me that both of you have had a difficult time coping with the changes in your lives over the past year. Have you ever considered therapy for yourself?"
**D.** "I'd like to learn more about your perceptions of what is happening with your wife. When did you first begin to notice a change in her behavior?"

**10** After 2 weeks on the psychiatric unit, L. appears less depressed. She participates in unit activities, maintains a groomed appearance, and expresses a desire to go home so she can "get on with her life." How should the treatment team respond?

**A.** Continue to observe L. carefully and to monitor her progress
**B.** Discharge L. as soon as possible
**C.** Allow L. to leave the unit unescorted and to go home periodically
**D.** Discontinue L.'s suicide precautions

---

### SITUATION

---

*B., a 50-year-old stockbroker, is transferred to the psychiatric unit after treatment for a self-inflicted gunshot wound to the chest. Although he has recovered from the physical injury, he continues to express suicidal ideation. B. was recently divorced by his wife of*

*25 years, and he is estranged from his 24-year-old son and 22-year-old daughter.*

*Questions 11 to 17 refer to this situation.*

**11** Which action is the nurse's highest priority during the initial patient interview?

**A.** Asking B. about the nature of his suicide attempt and whether he still has an active plan for it
**B.** Allowing B. to talk about his son and daughter
**C.** Encouraging B. to discuss his medical and psychiatric history
**D.** Persuading B. to use more appropriate coping mechanisms

**12** B. asks the nurse, "What do I have to live for? My wife left me and my children hate me. I'm all alone." Which response is most therapeutic?

**A.** "You are a successful businessman. Don't you get satisfaction from your work?"
**B.** "Have you tried to contact your family since your accident?"
**C.** "What do *you* think you have to live for?"
**D.** "You sound so hopeless. Are you saying you think suicide is your only option?"

**13** B. is on constant one-to-one observation. He complains that he cannot sleep with someone sitting next to him, looking at him every minute. How should the nurse reply?

**A.** "You are on strict suicide precautions and must be observed at all times"
**B.** "Why don't you discuss this with your physician? Maybe he can assign someone to sit outside your room"
**C.** "Your treatment plan requires constant observation for your safety. Where in your room would you prefer the staff member to sit?"
**D.** "I can appreciate what you are saying. I would be uncomfortable in that situation, too"

**14** B. tells the nursing assistant assigned to one-to-one duty that he is having severe stomach pains, and he asks her to get the nurse quickly. The assistant leaves B. and goes to the nurse's station. How should the nurse respond?

**A.** Remind the assistant that constant observation means just that, and send her back to B. immediately
**B.** Go with the assistant to B.'s room immediately
**C.** Question the assistant's judgment about leaving B. unattended even for a brief time
**D.** Call the physician to check on B. immediately

**15** Later the same afternoon, the nurse speaks with the nursing assistant about leaving B. alone. The best teaching approach is to:

**A.** Ask the assistant how the situation could have been handled better
**B.** Demonstrate how to palpate the abdomen to assess for tenderness and pain
**C.** Review the procedures for constant observation and explore ways to handle similar situations
**D.** Discuss the seriousness and legal ramifications of such a lapse in security

**16** B. is taken off one-to-one observation and placed on 15-minute checks. One afternoon, he is found hanging in the shower. Attempts to resuscitate him are ineffective. When the staff meets to discuss B.'s suicide, the focus should be on:

**A.** Determining who is responsible for the lapse in security
**B.** Preparing B.'s chart for review by hospital officials
**C.** Deciding who will speak with the patient's family
**D.** Ventilating feelings and thoroughly reviewing the case

**17** Staff members meet with the patients to discuss B.'s suicide. The chief rationale for such a meeting is to:

**A.** Dispel rumors regarding B.'s death
**B.** Detect other patients' suicidal ideation
**C.** Help the patients to ventilate their feelings about B.
**D.** Reassure the patients about their own safety and protection

---

### SITUATION

---

*J., age 57, is taken to the emergency department by two police officers after he tried to cut a supermarket manager with a piece of broken glass. He said he did this because he was just laid off from his job, which he held for 27 years. He also said his wife recently left him after 25 years of marriage because of his alcohol abuse and the physical abuse he inflicted on her when he was drunk. In the emergency department, he becomes verbally abusive to nursing staff members and demands to be released. When asked to be seated so the nurse can take his blood pressure, he throws a chair across the room. Four staff members are needed to control and restrain him.*

*J. is admitted to the psychiatric unit, placed in seclusion, and given haloperidol (Haldol) 5 mg I.M. After 1¹/₂ hours, he appears calmer and is released from seclusion. Although still angry, he is able to control himself from becoming physically or verbally abusive. He apologizes for his behavior and says that he hopes he did not hurt anyone.*

*Questions 18 to 24 refer to this situation.*

---

**18** Which response to J.'s apology is most therapeutic?

**A.** "We are here to help you. We understand that you didn't mean to hurt us"
**B.** "Let's see how well you can control yourself from now on"
**C.** "It's fortunate no one was hurt. It will not be necessary to use restraints as long as you can control your behavior"
**D.** "It was frightening and very dangerous. It is unpleasant to have to restrain someone"

---

**19** Based on J.'s history, reason for admission, and behavior in the emergency department, the nurse records that the patient has a *Potential for violence directed at others*. Which goal is most appropriate for this nursing diagnostic category?

**A.** The patient will verbalize anger rather than physically strike out
**B.** The patient will not strike out more than once per day
**C.** The patient will be placed in seclusion whenever he threatens anyone verbally or physically
**D.** The patient will not verbalize anger or strike out at anyone

**20** J. refuses his 5:00 p.m. 10-mg dose of haloperidol P.O. He states, "I'm in control now. I don't need any drugs." The nurse's response to J. should be based on the understanding that the patient:

**A.** Has the right to refuse treatment
**B.** Is potentially violent and must be medicated
**C.** Can be given haloperidol intramuscularly instead of orally
**D.** Must receive haloperidol at regular intervals to ensure the drug's effectiveness

**21** The nurse's initial priority when dealing with an assaultive or homicidal patient is to:

**A.** Keep the patient away from others and under one-to-one supervision
**B.** Restore the patient's self-control and prevent further loss of control
**C.** Allow the patient to act out his frustrations, then establish a line of communication
**D.** Clear the area of objects that might harm the patient or others

**22** One afternoon, the nurse hears J. yelling in the dayroom. He begins pushing chairs into the wall and swings at other patients with a pool cue. The nurse should intervene by:

**A.** Administering a fast-acting sedative, as ordered
**B.** Telling the patient to go to his room
**C.** Restraining the patient, then calling for assistance
**D.** Following the initial steps of the planned team approach

**23** J. continues to swing the pool cue wildly. Which approach is safest in this situation?

**A.** Approaching the patient as a team while holding a mattress and gently backing him toward a wall
**B.** Using chairs or other objects as safety barriers while approaching the patient
**C.** Keeping away from the patient until he puts the pool cue down
**D.** Calling hospital security to subdue the patient

**24** Which nursing intervention is most important when restraining a violent patient?

**A.** Reviewing hospital policy regarding how long the patient can be restrained
**B.** Preparing a PRN dose of the patient's psychotropic medication
**C.** Checking that the restraints have been applied correctly
**D.** Asking the patient if he needs to use the bathroom or is thirsty

## Answer sheet

A B C D
1 ○○○○
2 ○○○○
3 ○○○○
4 ○○○○
5 ○○○○
6 ○○○○
7 ○○○○
8 ○○○○
9 ○○○○
10 ○○○○
11 ○○○○
12 ○○○○
13 ○○○○
14 ○○○○
15 ○○○○
16 ○○○○
17 ○○○○
18 ○○○○
19 ○○○○
20 ○○○○
21 ○○○○
22 ○○○○
23 ○○○○
24 ○○○○

# Answers and rationales

**1** Correct answer—**C**

Mental health laws in most states set specific guidelines about the use of restraints. Most states allow restraints to be used if the patient presents a danger to himself or others. This danger must be reevaluated every few hours. If the patient is still a danger, restraints can be used until the violent behavior abates. No standing orders for restraints are allowed, and restraints are permitted only until "more humane" methods, such as sedatives, become effective. Violent patients who are intoxicated by drugs or alcohol present a problem because they usually cannot be sedated until the drug or alcohol is metabolized. In such cases, restraints may be needed for a longer period, but the patient must be closely observed. Obtaining consent is not always possible, especially when the patient's violent behavior results from psychosis, such as paranoid schizophrenia.

**2** Correct answer—**B**

A patient at highest risk for suicide is one who plans a violent death (for example, by gunshot, jumping off a bridge, or hanging), has a specific plan (for example, after his wife leaves for work), and has the means readily available (for example, a rifle hidden in the garage). A patient who gives away possessions, thinks about death, or talks about wanting to die or attempting suicide is considered at a lower risk for suicide because his behavior typically serves to alert others that he is contemplating suicide and that he wishes to be helped.

**3** Correct answer—**A**

Studies of those who commit suicide reveal the following high-risk groups: adolescents; men over age 45; previous suicide attempters; divorced, widowed, or separated persons; professionals, such as physicians, dentists, and attorneys; students; unemployed persons; persons who are depressed, delusional, or hallucinating; alcohol or substance abusers; and persons who live in urban areas. Although women attempt suicide more often than men do, they typically choose less lethal means and are therefore less likely to succeed in their attempts.

**4** Correct answer—**A**

Suicidal persons have certain common characteristics, regardless of the factors that brought them to a suicidal state. One of the most common features is ambivalence—an internal struggle between self-preserving and self-destructive forces. These doubts are expressed when persons threaten or attempt suicide and then try to get help to be saved. When the possible consequences of suicide are discussed with such persons, they often describe life-related outcomes, such as relief from an unhappy situation. Many people may consider suicide as an alternative to their present circumstances, but they may not have considered the implications of not living. Remorse and anger may be associated with depression, but these feelings are not universally present in suicidal persons. A psychotic individual may or may not have suicidal tendencies.

**5** Correct answer—**D**

One of the nurse's primary responsibilities when assessing a suicidal patient is to determine whether the patient has a specific plan, what the plan entails, and whether the patient has the means available to act on the plan. A patient with a specific plan and access to lethal means is at a higher risk for suicide than one who has a vague plan and no available lethal method. Only after making such determinations should the nurse assure the patient that the staff will protect her from self-injury. Exploring the patient's feelings about her relationship with her husband and her feelings of failure will follow as part of the therapeutic relationship. Persuading a despondent, suicidal patient to think about how lucky she is to have survived would further increase her feelings of failure.

**6** Correct answer—**B**

L. must not be left alone at this time. She has made a serious suicide attempt and is continuing to verbalize suicidal intent. While the nursing staff collaborates on how best to implement suicide precautions, a nurse or nursing assistant who has been instructed on the necessary observations and appropriate interventions should remain with the patient to observe her on a one-to-one basis. Although a sedative may help to calm the patient and reduce her suicidal ideation, the nurses still need to ensure the patient's safety while obtaining the medication order. Restraints should not be used unless all other available means to protect the patient from injury have failed. Although a psychiatric consultation is appropriate to plan effective care, the nurse's first responsibility is to protect the patient from self-injury.

## 7 Correct answer—A

Visitors and telephone calls usually are restricted only when requested by the patient or when a specific therapeutic reason exists (for example, if such interaction would be too stressful for the patient). These restrictions usually are lifted once the patient can cope with the feelings generated by such encounters. General and psychiatric hospitals should have clearly stated suicide precautions as part of their policy manuals. Such precautions typically include removing all dangerous objects, such as razors, glass, scissors, electrical cords, and belts from the patient's reach; searching the patient's belongings and visitors' packages and surveying the room and surrounding areas for potentially dangerous objects; securing windows; and assigning the patient a room near the nurse's station. The nurse must explain the suicide precautions to the patient, staff members, and all visitors who have contact with the patient. This explanation is necessary to prevent someone from inadvertently providing the patient with some means (for example, matches, a nail file, or a belt) to carry out suicidal ideas.

## 8 Correct answer—A

Because L. has been transferred to a new environment with new staff members, maintaining—if not increasing—the level of suicide precautions is wise. The precautions can be modified after the health care team has had a chance to evaluate the patient's suicidal ideation. Being on a locked psychiatric unit is not in itself enough protection against self-destructive behavior. Suicidal patients who are actively suicidal (expressing suicidal ideas and having definite plans of action) should never be left alone. Suicide precautions should be eased only when the suicide risk has decreased and the patient no longer discusses a definite suicide plan.

## 9 Correct answer—D

Assessing Mr. C.'s perceptions of his wife's problems and learning when he first began to notice a change in her behavior are important for two reasons: the nurse needs to understand Mr. C.'s perception of the situation to respond therapeutically, and Mr. C. may be able to provide some background about his wife's difficulties. Although the patient's problems may be related to her husband's job loss, the nurse should avoid making Mr. C. feel defensive by blaming him for his wife's actions. Mr. C. is asking for help in understanding the crisis he and his wife are facing. The nurse needs to learn more from him before offering guidance about how to approach his wife, her needs, or his possible need for therapy.

## 10 Correct answer—A

The treatment team must continue to observe L. carefully and to monitor her progress. Commonly, suicidal patients are ambivalent about living and dying and may appear less depressed once they have decided to kill themselves and have formulated a plan. Allowing increased freedom, discontinuing precautions, and planning for discharge should be done only after the patient has been thoroughly evaluated by the entire treatment team.

## 11 Correct answer—A

The nurse's highest priority during the initial interview is determining whether the patient still has an active plan to commit suicide so that she can assess the likelihood of another suicide attempt. After evaluating this information, the nurse should explore the patient's feelings of inadequacy in coping with the immediate and chronic stresses in his life, his level of hope, and his view of the intolerableness of the situation. Such exploration enables the nurse to formulate nursing diagnoses and an effective plan of care.

## 12 Correct answer—D

When a patient expresses hopelessness and suicidal intentions, the nurse must ask him directly about possible suicidal plans. Such questioning enables the nurse to assess the patient's level of suicide risk and to tell the patient that she recognizes his distress and wants to help. Even more important, it lets the patient know that talk about his feelings is acceptable. Denying the patient's feelings by commenting on his success as a businessman is nonempathetic and distances the nurse from the patient. Referring to the suicide attempt as an "accident" is nontherapeutic because it denies the patient's desperate situation. A despondent patient would find it too difficult to identify what he has to live for.

## 13 Correct answer—C

The nurse should respond honestly and empathically to B.'s complaint. She can accomplish both objectives by explaining the reason for constant observation and by working with the patient to identify a place for the staff member to sit that will meet the patient's protection and comfort needs. Telling the patient that he is on suicide precautions and must be observed at all times places blame on the patient for his situation and is not an empathic response. Because constant observation means that the patient must always be in clear view, having the staff member sit outside the room is unacceptable. Mere acknowledgment of the patient's feelings is nontherapeutic because it offers no solution to the problem.

## 14 Correct answer—B

Because B. should not be left alone at any time while on one-to-one constant observation, the nurse should accompany the nursing assistant immediately to B.'s room to assess the situation and ensure his safety. The nurse should not waste time reviewing constant observation procedures, discussing the assistant's judgment, or calling the physician. Such actions may be done after she has had time to assess the patient's status.

## 15 Correct answer—C

The most effective teaching method in this situation would incorporate a review of the procedures and rationale for constant observation of a suicidal patient. After reinforcing previous learning, the nurse can help the nursing assistant to identify more appropriate responses that could be taken in a similar situation, such as calling for assistance from the patient's room, bringing the patient to the nurse, using the call system or phone, or asking another patient to summon help. Asking the assistant to identify alternative ways of handling the situation may be helpful but would not ensure her understanding of critical aspects associated with institutional procedures, including the legal ramifications of leaving a patient unattended. Teaching abdominal palpation would be inappropriate, since performing a physical assessment is part of the nurse's, not assistant's, responsibility.

## 16 Correct answer—D

After a patient commits suicide, staff members must meet to discuss the event and to ventilate their feelings, which may range from grief, guilt, and anger to failure and inadequacy. Meeting together provides an opportunity to give and receive support. A thorough and careful case review may identify missed clues or errors of judgment in the patient's treatment, which could help protect other patients in the future. Hospital authorities will conduct an in-depth case review to determine any liability on the part of staff members. Every patient's chart is an important legal document and should be kept up to date and ready for review at all times. The patient's physician, not a nursing staff member, is responsible for talking with the patient's family.

## 17 Correct answer—D

When a patient attempts or commits suicide on the unit, staff members must hold a meeting with the patients to discuss the event. Many patients become frightened and believe that their safety is compromised or that they are in danger. They may be afraid that the staff cannot protect them from their own dangerous thoughts and impulses. Therefore, the chief reason for the meeting is to reassure the patients that staff members can and will protect them. The meeting also can serve to dispel rumors about B.'s death and may lead to a discussion of other patients' self-destructive thoughts. Patients also may express their feelings about B. and his death. Regardless of the tone the meeting takes, staff members must send a clear message that the patients will be protected.

## 18 Correct answer—C

The most therapeutic response to J.'s apology should incorporate a realistic statement acknowledging, in a nonpunitive but serious manner, the possible consequences of his violent behavior. The nurse also should set clear limits by describing the expected behavior and the consequences the patient will face if he again loses control. Violent behavior is dangerous to both the patient and others and should not be excused or made light of by saying "I know you didn't mean to hurt us..." or "Let's see how well you control yourself from now on." Such statements neither reinforce the risk of violently acting out nor define limits for future behavior. Restraining a patient is unpleasant for all concerned, but disclosing this information to the patient without addressing the dangerousness of his behavior and reinforcing what is expected of him is insufficient.

## 19 Correct answer—A

Verbalizing angry feelings instead of physically striking out is an appropriate treatment goal for this patient. J. needs an outlet for his anger, and as long as he does not express threats of violence, verbalizing his angry feelings is an acceptable way to discharge his emotions. Striking out is an unacceptable behavior at any time. Placing the patient in seclusion in response to his threats is a nursing intervention, not a therapeutic goal.

## 20 Correct answer—A

When formulating her response, the nurse must recognize that the patient has the right to refuse treatment, including medications. She also should be knowledgeable about state laws and institutional policies regarding this issue. Generally, patients can be treated against their will only in emergencies in which the safety of the patient or others is threatened. A potential for violence is not a sufficient reason to medicate a patient against his will. Even though haloperidol (Haldol) can be given intramuscularly instead of orally, the nurse cannot forcibly administer an intramuscular injection to a patient who refuses treatment but poses no immediate physical threat. Although effective blood levels of haloperidol are achieved through regular dosing, this consideration does not override that of the patient's right to refuse treatment.

## 21 Correct answer—B

The priority nursing intervention in response to an assaultive or homicidal patient is to maintain safety by restoring the patient's self-control and preventing further loss of control. The nurse must quickly assess the situation, then attempt to restore control through interpersonal interventions, such as using a team approach, removing the patient from the situation, encouraging verbalization, setting limits, and talking the patient down—speaking in a calm, well-modulated voice and providing verbal support and reassurance that the patient will not be harmed and will not be permitted to hurt himself or others. If such measures fail to control the patient, other interventions, such as seclusion, medication, or restraint, may be necessary. Acting out violently is dangerous to the patient and others and must be controlled. Unless the patient is in seclusion, clearing the area of potentially harmful objects is unrealistic because the staff or other patients may need access to those objects. Also, one of the goals of therapy is to help the patient develop self-control and learn to coexist with others.

## 22 Correct answer—D

The treatment team should have a plan for dealing with violent or potentially violent patients, which should be taught to all staff members and reviewed periodically. The plan should clearly de-

fine the approach and specify roles for each team member. A show
of force by all team members is sometimes sufficient to influence
the patient to cooperate. The best plan involves a team leader and
four or five additional staff members who are each assigned a specific task, such as securing the patient's left leg, right leg, left arm,
and right arm. The leader typically serves as the spokesperson for
the team.

Approaching the patient to administer medication or telling
him to go to his room may be unsafe without the support and
backup of other team members. The nurse should never attempt
to approach or restrain a violent patient by herself.

## 23 Correct answer—A

The patient's behavior is clearly dangerous and must be stopped
before someone is injured. An organized plan to ensure the safety
of the patient and the staff is essential. While the patient is striking
out, staff members, through a team approach, can be protected
from injury by using a mattress as a shield. Unlike chairs or other
objects, the mattress provides padding to protect the patient as he
is slowly backed toward the wall and restrained. Trained psychiatric staff members, not hospital security, should handle the restraint
of a psychiatric patient.

## 24 Correct answer—C

The nurse must determine whether the restraints have been applied correctly. This assessment ensures that the patient's circula-
tion and respiration are not restricted and that adequate padding
has been used. The nurse should document carefully the patient's
response and status after being restrained. All staff members involved in restraining patients should be aware of hospital policy
before using restraints. If PRN medication is ordered, it should be
given before restraints are in place and with the assistance of other
team members. The nurse should attend to the patient's elimination and hydration needs after the patient is properly restrained.

# CHAPTER 7

# Maladaptive Behavior

## Questions

### SITUATION

*T., a 38-year-old father of three, voluntarily admits himself to the substance abuse unit. He admits to drinking a quart or more of vodka each day and to occasional cocaine use. His job is in jeopardy, and his wife has threatened to leave him.*

*Questions 1 to 10 refer to this situation.*

**1** Medication orders for T. most likely will include:

**A.** Chlordiazepoxide (Librium), multivitamins, thiamine, and folic acid
**B.** Vitamins B and C and phenytoin (Dilantin)
**C.** Vitamins A and E and haloperidol (Haldol)
**D.** Vitamin B, acetaminophen (Tylenol), and a laxative

**2** Later that afternoon, T. begins to show signs of alcohol withdrawal. Early signs of this condition include:

**A.** Vomiting, diarrhea, and bradycardia
**B.** Dehydration, temperature above 101° F (38.3° C), and pruritus
**C.** Hypertension, diaphoresis, and convulsions
**D.** Diaphoresis, tremors, and nervousness

**3** Which assessment finding is most consistent with alcohol withdrawal?

**A.** Pulse rate of 120 to 140 beats/minute
**B.** Pulse rate of 50 to 60 beats/minute
**C.** Blood pressure of 100/70 mm Hg
**D.** Blood pressure of 200/100 mm Hg

**4** T. begins to experience alcoholic hallucinosis. The best nursing intervention at this time is to:

**A.** Keep the patient restrained in bed
**B.** Check the patient's blood pressure every 15 minutes and offer him juices
**C.** Provide a quiet environment and administer medication as needed
**D.** Restrain the patient and check his blood pressure every 30 minutes

**5** T. experiences illusions at night. He cries out, "There's something in the corner." The nurse can help T. by:

**A.** Permitting him to stay up all night in the dayroom
**B.** Staying with him all night to provide support
**C.** Leaving a light on in his room
**D.** Allowing him to sit with her in the nurse's station

**6** T. begins to show paranoid behavior. He states, "I know that the neighbors are after me for beating my wife when I'm drunk." Before responding, the nurse should recognize that the patient is exhibiting a thought disorder called:

**A.** Nihilistic delusion
**B.** Delusion of persecution
**C.** Delusion of grandeur
**D.** Idea of reference

**7** While T. is in a paranoid state, the nurse finds interacting with him frustrating. Establishing and maintaining a therapeutic relationship is extremely difficult at this time because:

**A.** A paranoid patient typically views everyone as conspiring against him
**B.** An alcoholic patient typically mistrusts others
**C.** An alcoholic patient typically thinks that others take advantage of him
**D.** A paranoid patient typically becomes dependent on others quickly

**8** The physician prescribes disulfiram (Antabuse) for T. Which medications should the nurse instruct T. to avoid while he is taking this drug?

**A.** Antacids
**B.** Aspirin and acetaminophen
**C.** Most cough syrups
**D.** Blood pressure medications

**9** T. has been on the unit for 1 month. One afternoon after visiting hours, he becomes extremely loud and talkative in the dayroom. On physical examination, the nurse notes tachycardia, blood pressure of 150/90 mm Hg, and dilated pupils. The nurse suspects:

A. Alcohol intoxication
B. Alcohol withdrawal syndrome
C. Cocaine intoxication
D. Cocaine withdrawal syndrome

**10** T.'s wife expresses concern about T.'s ability to maintain his recovery from substance abuse after discharge. The nurse suggests that she consider:

A. Alcoholics Anonymous
B. Al-Anon
C. Psychotherapy
D. Trial separation from her husband

## SITUATION

*J., a 25-year-old man, is hospitalized for treatment of fractures of the right femur and right humerus. These injuries were the result of a motorcycle accident. Police suspect that J. was intoxicated at the time of the accident. Laboratory tests reveal a blood alcohol level of 0.2% (200 mg/dl). J. later admits that he has been drinking heavily for years.*

*Questions 11 to 17 refer to this situation.*

**11** After J.'s fractures are set in the emergency department, he is assigned to a semiprivate room on the medical-surgical unit. The nurse who admitted J. to the unit prepares to conduct a complete patient assessment. Which question is most important to ask during the history-taking session?

A. "How often do you drink alcohol?"
B. "When was your last drink?"
C. "Did you realize you were intoxicated while driving?"
D. "Why did you drink?"

**12** Three days after admission, J. becomes nauseated and begins to shake slightly. His pulse rate is 110 beats/minute, and his blood pressure is 170/100 mm Hg. All of the following nursing interventions are appropriate at this time *except:*

   **A.** Administering phenytoin 100 mg I.V. stat
   **B.** Arranging to move J. to a private room
   **C.** Calling the physician to report the findings
   **D.** Reassuring J. that he is not alone and will be cared for

**13** After receiving a sedative, J. begins to yell, "Get those hairy spiders off me. They're crawling all over me." The nurse realizes that J. is probably experiencing:

   **A.** A reaction to the sedative
   **B.** A schizophrenic episode
   **C.** Symptoms of alcohol withdrawal delirium
   **D.** A psychological reaction to the casts on his arm and leg

**14** How should the nurse respond to J.'s hallucination?

   **A.** Pretend to kill the spiders
   **B.** Encourage him to rest, then leave him alone
   **C.** Remain with him, providing frequent orientation and reassurance
   **D.** Give him coffee and keep him ambulatory with the assistance of two aides until he becomes calm

**15** The nurse realizes that alcohol withdrawal delirium should be viewed as:

   **A.** A commonplace reaction to alcohol withdrawal that subsides uneventfully
   **B.** A serious physical response with potential for death
   **C.** An unusual, frightening, but relatively safe withdrawal symptom
   **D.** An avoidable emotional reaction to the loss a person feels when he stops drinking

**16** During his hospitalization, J. periodically complains of tingling and numbness in his hands and feet. The nurse realizes that these symptoms probably are caused by:

**A.** Thiamine deficiency
**B.** Acetate accumulation
**C.** Triglyceride buildup
**D.** Low serum potassium levels

**17** One week after discharge, J. is brought to the emergency department by his father, who suspects that J. overdosed during a party. J. is sleeping soundly, his pupils are constricted, and no odor of alcohol is on his breath. Besides notifying J.'s physician, the nurse should immediately:

**A.** Obtain cloth restraints and observe J. for psychotic behavior
**B.** Obtain an order for a central nervous system depressant to prevent alcohol withdrawal delirium and monitor J.'s blood pressure every 15 minutes
**C.** Obtain an order for a sedative and remain alert to the possibility of agitation
**D.** Obtain an order for a narcotic antagonist and continuously monitor J.'s respiration and other vital signs

## SITUATION

*B., a 23-year-old unmarried man, is remanded by the courts for psychiatric treatment. He has a police record dating to his early teenage years that includes delinquency, running away, auto theft, vandalism, and other infractions. He dropped out of school at age 16 and has been living on his own since then.*

*Questions 18 to 26 refer to this situation.*

**18** B.'s history suggests maladaptive coping, which is associated with which type of personality disorder?

**A.** Antisocial
**B.** Borderline
**C.** Obsessive-compulsive
**D.** Narcissistic

**19** During the admission interview, B. boasts to the nurse that he has "knocked up" (made pregnant) at least three girls in the past year. When the nurse asks what responsibility he feels for this, he laughingly replies, "Nothing. It's not my problem. I have my needs." B.'s response shows evidence of:

A. A high self-esteem and a strong self-concept
B. Anxiety
C. Sexual addiction
D. An inability to form long-term emotional attachments

**20** The nurse asks B. to remove the heavy quilted shirt he is wearing so she can take his blood pressure. B. replies, "I'll strip naked for you, baby." Which response is most appropriate?

A. "You're very attractive, but I am a nurse, not one of your girlfriends"
B. "I only need access to your arm. Removing your shirt will be fine"
C. "Maybe I should call one of the male aides to help you control yourself"
D. "First, I'm not your baby. And second, you wouldn't be the first naked man I've seen"

**21** A primary focus of B.'s treatment plan will be to help him:

A. Establish mature relationships with women
B. Recognize and observe limits when interacting with others
C. Express feelings of remorse about past behaviors
D. Choose a stable career or occupation

**22** B.'s care plan should include:

A. Administering medication to prevent acting out
B. Providing flexibility in his daily schedule to avoid confrontations over authority
C. Restricting him to his room with limited access to other more vulnerable patients
D. Providing a structured environment and setting clear limits

**23** One morning, B. approaches the nurse and asks to be allowed to go to the coffee shop. He says, "Because I've been so good this week, I now have privileges." The nurse has just returned from a week-long vacation and has not yet seen his report. How should she respond to B.?

**A.** "I'm glad to hear you've been following the rules. Remember to sign out before you leave"
**B.** "I doubt if things could have changed so much in a week. You'll have to wait until later"
**C.** "I've been off for a week. I'll have to check on your privilege status first"
**D.** "I'd really like to believe you, but I can't. I'm sorry, but I have to check first"

**24** One of the patients on the unit reports that B. has been taking advantage of the other patients. He states that B. has been "borrowing" money, cigarettes, and clothing without returning the items or reciprocating the favor. The best way to approach B. about this reported behavior is to:

**A.** Say nothing to him and have staff members observe him for such behaviors
**B.** Confront B. on a one-to-one basis
**C.** Ask the patients involved to confront B. in a community meeting
**D.** Limit B.'s interactions with other patients by restricting him to his room

**25** The staff members begin to notice a relationship developing between B. and a 17-year-old female patient, who have been seen holding hands and dancing seductively while listening to the radio. Staff members are concerned about possible sexual acting out by both patients. Which is the best approach to this situation?

**A.** Continuing to observe both patients closely without directly confronting them
**B.** Counseling both patients individually about safe sexual practices
**C.** Talking with both patients about the rules regarding physical contact
**D.** Telling B. that he cannot spend any time with the other patient

**26** One afternoon during an art group, B. begins berating the work of several other patients, saying "That looks like something painted by a 2-year-old. What a piece of garbage" and "You guys must really be nuts if that's the best you can do." The group leader warns B. that he should keep such comments to himself or he will have to leave the group. B. laughs and says, "I'm the only one who knows what I'm doing. If I leave, you'd be left with zombies." How should the group leader respond?

**A.** Ignore B.'s comments because he is just testing the group leader's authority
**B.** Ask the group members what they think of B.'s work
**C.** Encourage the group members to tell B. how they feel about his remarks
**D.** Tell B. that he must leave the group

## SITUATION

*M., age 24, goes to the community mental health clinic because she feels depressed and abandoned and does not know what to do with her life. Her history reveals that she dropped out of high school 6 months before graduation and has worked at numerous clerical jobs since then. She claims that she typically quits after only a short time on the job because the people do not seem to like her and do not teach her what to do. Last week, her boyfriend broke up with her after she drove his car into a tree after an argument. The initial diagnosis is borderline personality disorder.*

*Questions 27 and 28 refer to this situation.*

**27** Which symptoms support a diagnosis of borderline personality disorder?

**A.** Lack of self-esteem, strong dependency needs, and impulsive behavior
**B.** Flat affect, social withdrawal, and unusual dress
**C.** Suspiciousness, hypervigilance, and emotional coldness
**D.** Insensitivity to others, sexual acting out, and violence

**28** One afternoon, M. becomes angry in the clinic waiting room after being told that the nurse will be a half hour late because of an emergency. When the nurse arrives, M. shouts, "I never did like you. I want to be assigned to someone else." Which response by the nurse is best?

A. "Waiting for someone who's late can be frustrating. Let's talk about what you're feeling right now"
B. "I'm sorry that you had to wait, but I needed to attend to an emergency"
C. "I understand that you are angry and upset, but don't you think you're overreacting by requesting another nurse?"
D. "I'm sorry that you feel we cannot continue to work together. I'll request for you to be reassigned to another nurse"

## SITUATION

*D., age 21, is admitted to the hospital for detoxification from heroin. He is unmarried and lives in an abandoned building with friends who also use drugs and frequently share needles. This is his third admission to the detoxification unit this year.*

*Questions 29 to 32 refer to this situation.*

**29** How long after the last dose of heroin should the nurse expect to note early symptoms of heroin withdrawal?

A. 1 to 2 hours
B. 4 to 6 hours
C. 8 to 12 hours
D. 48 to 72 hours

**30** D. is admitted to the unit from the emergency department, where the admitting physician prescribed methadone hydrochloride (Dolophine) 40 mg P.O. q6h. The nurse should:

A. Administer the medication as ordered
B. Dissolve the medication in a small amount of juice before administering it
C. Question the patient about his drug history
D. Call the physician to discuss the order

**31** The nurse should follow universal precautions as defined by the Centers for Disease Control when caring for patients such as D., who is at high risk for:

**A.** Endocarditis and septicemia
**B.** Tuberculosis
**C.** Syphilis
**D.** Acquired immunodeficiency syndrome

**32** D. tells the nurse that he is considering entering a residential therapeutic community for drug treatment. He asks her what is involved in such a program. The nurse should respond by saying:

**A.** "Such programs try to help people abstain from drugs and learn new coping skills. They usually require a 12- to 18-month commitment"
**B.** "The programs are essentially self-help groups in which recovered addicts help other persons who want to recover from drug addiction"
**C.** "The programs use various treatment modalities, such as methadone maintenance, psychotherapy, and group therapy, to help people abstain from drugs"
**D.** "Such programs are conducted on an outpatient basis to allow people to maintain their jobs and family responsibilities while undergoing treatment"

# Answer sheet

| | A B C D | | A B C D |
|---|---|---|---|
| 1 | ○○○○ | 31 | ○○○○ |
| 2 | ○○○○ | 32 | ○○○○ |
| 3 | ○○○○ | | |
| 4 | ○○○○ | | |
| 5 | ○○○○ | | |
| 6 | ○○○○ | | |
| 7 | ○○○○ | | |
| 8 | ○○○○ | | |
| 9 | ○○○○ | | |
| 10 | ○○○○ | | |
| 11 | ○○○○ | | |
| 12 | ○○○○ | | |
| 13 | ○○○○ | | |
| 14 | ○○○○ | | |
| 15 | ○○○○ | | |
| 16 | ○○○○ | | |
| 17 | ○○○○ | | |
| 18 | ○○○○ | | |
| 19 | ○○○○ | | |
| 20 | ○○○○ | | |
| 21 | ○○○○ | | |
| 22 | ○○○○ | | |
| 23 | ○○○○ | | |
| 24 | ○○○○ | | |
| 25 | ○○○○ | | |
| 26 | ○○○○ | | |
| 27 | ○○○○ | | |
| 28 | ○○○○ | | |
| 29 | ○○○○ | | |
| 30 | ○○○○ | | |

# Answers and rationales

**1** Correct answer—**A**

Chlordiazepoxide (Librium), multivitamins, thiamine, and folic acid are the medications of choice for a newly admitted substance abuser. Chlordiazepoxide helps prevent seizures, and multivitamins, thiamine, and folic acid help prevent further neurologic degeneration associated with alcoholism. Other vitamins, such as D, K, and A, may be ordered after the physician further evaluates the patient's nutritional status. Acetaminophen (Tylenol) may exacerbate liver problems and therefore is used cautiously in substance abusers, who commonly have liver disease. Liver damage can be caused by cirrhosis and alcoholic hepatitis or viral hepatitis resulting from injected drugs. Phenytoin (Dilantin), haloperidol (Haldol), and laxatives are not used to treat substance abuse.

**2** Correct answer—**D**

Alcohol withdrawal syndrome includes alcohol withdrawal, alcoholic hallucinosis, and alcohol withdrawal delirium (formerly delirium tremens). Signs of alcohol withdrawal include diaphoresis, tremors, and nervousness, as well as nausea, vomiting, malaise, increased blood pressure and pulse rate, sleep disturbance, and irritability. Although diarrhea may be an early sign, tachycardia—not bradycardia—is associated with alcohol withdrawal. Dehydration and elevated temperature may be expected, but a temperature above 101° F (38.3° C) indicates an infection rather than alcohol withdrawal. Pruritus is not a common complaint. If withdrawal symptoms remain untreated, seizures may be seen later.

**3** Correct answer—**A**

Tachycardia—a pulse rate of 120 to 140 beats/minute—is a common sign of alcohol withdrawal. Blood pressure may be labile throughout withdrawal, fluctuating at different stages. Hypertension typically is noted in early withdrawal; hypotension, although rare during the early withdrawal stages, may occur in later stages. It is associated with cardiovascular collapse and most often seen in patients who do not receive treatment. The nurse should carefully monitor the patient's vital signs throughout the entire alcohol withdrawal process.

**4** Correct answer—**C**

Alcoholic hallucinosis typically occurs within the first 48 to 72 hours after drinking stops. It is characterized by auditory hallucinations, delusions, and clouding of consciousness. These symptoms are best treated by providing a quiet environment to reduce stimuli and by administering central nervous system depressants, such as chlordiazepoxide, diazepam (Valium), phenobarbital (Barbita), or paraldehyde (Paral), in dosages that control symptoms without causing oversedation. This combination helps control the patient's symptoms and agitation, which can last for a few hours to several days. Although bed rest is indicated, restraining the patient is unnecessary unless he is a danger to himself or others. Restraints can increase a patient's agitation and make him feel trapped and helpless when hallucinating. Offering juice is appropriate, but checking the patient's blood pressure every 15 minutes would interrupt his rest. Blood pressure should be checked every 2 hours to avoid overstimulating the patient.

**5** Correct answer—**C**

Leaving a light on in T.'s room can help prevent visual distortion. The light should decrease shadows in the room and lessen his illusions. T.'s need for rest is not met by allowing him to stay up all night in the dayroom or at the nurse's station. Unless T. is in need of one-to-one supervision, the nurse need not stay with him all night.

**6** Correct answer—**B**

T. is displaying delusion of persecution, the belief that he is being unfairly harassed or persecuted by others. Nihilistic delusion is a type of delusion in which a person denies his existence or some part of himself, such as "I am dead" or "I have no stomach." Delusion of grandeur is a type of delusion in which a person falsely believes that he is extremely important, powerful, or rich. Idea of reference describes the thought pattern of a person who believes that events in the environment or the actions of others are related to him—for example, "Everyone is looking at me" or "When I get to the corner, the streetlight will turn red." Patients with delusions of persecution commonly exhibit ideas of reference.

## 7 Correct answer—A

T. is exhibiting paranoid behavior, which includes delusions of persecution. A patient with this thought disorder views others as a threat, making interaction difficult because he typically tries to push people away to protect himself. The nurse must overcome her frustration by using a consistent approach to establishing a trusting relationship. Generalizations about the personality traits of alcoholic patients rarely are accurate or helpful in planning interventions to meet their needs. Paranoid patients typically have difficulty trusting, and thus do not quickly become dependent on others.

## 8 Correct answer—C

A patient who is taking disulfiram (Antabuse) must avoid alcohol in any form or he may experience a severe adverse reaction. The nurse should advise the patient that most cough syrups contain alcohol. She also should advise him to avoid foods containing alcohol, skin lotions, and alchohol-based shaving creams. To help ensure compliance with these instructions, the nurse should give the patient a list of substances to avoid as well as teach him to read labels and question whether food prepared in restaurants contains alcohol. The patient should wear a medical alert bracelet or tag or carry an ID card indicating that he is taking disulfiram. A patient receiving disulfiram who ingests even small amounts of alcohol may experience flushed skin, pounding headache, weakness, dizziness, nausea, vomiting, tachycardia, chest pain, dyspnea, hypotension, blurred vision, and confusion. If large amounts of alcohol are consumed, the reaction can lead to respiratory and cardiac collapse, unconsciousness, convulsions, and even death.

Aspirin and acetaminophen are detoxified in the liver and should be used cautiously in patients who may have liver damage. Patients taking prescribed antihypertensive medication should not discontinue these drugs without a physician's permission. Doing so can lead to additional medical problems, such as a possible cerebrovascular accident. Other drugs, such as antacids, can be taken, but the patient should clear their use with a physician.

## 9 Correct answer—C

The nurse should suspect cocaine intoxication rather than alcohol withdrawal or intoxication. Symptoms indicative of cocaine intoxication include increased heart rate and blood pressure, dilated pupils, sweating, chills, nausea and vomiting, talkativeness, elation, increased sense of well-being, and agitation. Alcohol intoxication is characterized by slurred speech, incoordination, ataxia, nystagmus, flushed face, impaired judgment, and fighting. Alcohol withdrawal syndrome, which would be seen within 1 week of the patient's cessation of drinking, is evidenced by clouding of consciousness, illusions, visual hallucinations, incoherent speech, agitation, and increased blood pressure. Cocaine withdrawal syndrome has not yet been described; however, a patient withdrawing from cocaine typically experiences depression, fatigue, and anxiety.

## 10 Correct answer—B

Al-Anon is a self-help program that began as an offshoot of Alcoholics Anonymous (AA). It is a group for spouses, relatives, and friends of alcoholics who meet to share their experiences, strength, hope, and support. Al-Anon focuses not on the alcoholic patient but on the relatives and friends themselves and on improving their own lives through the 12 steps of the AA program. AA is a self-help group for the alcoholic person who wants to stop drinking. Psychotherapy would be appropriate if T.'s wife expresses a need for professional help. Decisions or suggestions regarding trial separation should come from T.'s wife. If she mentions the idea, the nurse should allow her to verbalize her feelings about it. The nurse should not make recommendations about separation because it shifts responsibility for the decision from T.'s wife to the nurse.

## 11 Correct answer—B

The nurse must determine when the patient last ingested alcohol so that interventions can be started to prevent alcohol withdrawal syndrome. If untreated, this syndrome can progress to alcoholic hallucinosis and alcohol withdrawal delirium, both of which are serious and life-threatening conditions. Although the nurse will need to obtain J.'s alcohol history (including types, amounts, and frequency of use), the priority at this time is to determine when alcohol was last ingested. Challenging the patient by asking if he knew he was intoxicated while driving or why he drinks would probably alienate him and hinder development of a therapeutic relationship.

**12** Correct answer—**A**

J. probably is experiencing early alcohol withdrawal. However, because he is not having seizures, he will not require phenytoin I.V. Moving J. to a private room to decrease stimuli, informing the physician of his status, and communicating reassurance and support are appropriate interventions because a patient going through withdrawal typically feels anxious and fearful.

**13** Correct answer—**C**

The patient has probably progressed to alcohol withdrawal delirium (formerly delirium tremens). Characteristic symptoms include tremors, rapid pulse, fever, and increased blood pressure; these symptoms tend to worsen over time. A patient in advanced alcohol withdrawal delirium typically experiences confusion, delusions, and hallucinations (auditory, visual, or tactile) and becomes extremely fearful. Additional physical complications of untreated alcohol withdrawal delirium include pneumonia and cardiac failure. The patient's medication and his casts are unlikely to cause such hallucinations. A patient experiencing a schizophrenic episode typically exhibits auditory, not visual or tactile, hallucinations.

**14** Correct answer—**C**

A disoriented and fearful patient who is experiencing distorted reality is at risk for injury, so the patient must not be left alone. The patient needs the supportive presence of the nurse to reassure, orient, and protect him from injury. Pretending to kill the spiders reinforces the hallucination and is not helpful. The caffeine in coffee, plus the added stimulation of walking with two nursing assistants, would increase—not decrease—the patient's agitation. A patient experiencing alcohol withdrawal delirium needs a quiet environment in order to rest.

**15** Correct answer—**B**

Alcohol withdrawal delirium is the physiologic result of withdrawing from alcohol. It is a serious condition that, if untreated, can result in death from cardiac or respiratory complications. Alcohol withdrawal delirium is not a common occurrence if the patient receives treatment. Because it can cause serious complications, alcohol withdrawal delirium is not a safe withdrawal symptom. The delirium is a physiologic response to the absence of alcohol, not an emotional reaction.

## 16 Correct answer—A

Numbness and tingling in the hands and feet are symptoms of peripheral polynephritis, which results from an inadequate intake of vitamin $B_1$ (thiamine) secondary to prolonged and excessive alcohol intake. Treatment includes reducing alcohol intake, correcting nutritional deficiencies through diet and vitamin supplements, and preventing such residual disabilities as foot and wrist drop. Acetate accumulation, triglyceride buildup, and low serum potassium levels are unrelated to J.'s symptoms.

## 17 Correct answer—D

Sound sleeping, constricted pupils, and the absence of alcohol odor on his breath suggest that J. ingested narcotics. Because non-obstructive respiratory failure is a potential complication of drug overdose, the nurse must continuously monitor the patient's respiration and vital signs. She also should make sure that oxygen and a narcotic antagonist, such as naloxone (Narcan), are available in case of respiratory depression. Since J. is not awake or agitated, restraints are unnecessary. No evidence of alcohol withdrawal syndrome or alcohol intoxication is present. The nurse's primary concern is the depressant effect of the narcotic overdose, not agitation.

## 18 Correct answer—A

B.'s history of delinquency, running away from home, vandalism, and dropping out of school are characteristic of someone with antisocial personality disorder. This maladaptive coping pattern is manifested by a disregard for societal norms of behavior and an inability to relate meaningfully to others. In borderline personality disorder, the person exhibits mood instability, poor self-image, identity disturbance, and labile affect. Obsessive-compulsive personality disorder is characterized by a preoccupation with impulses and thoughts that the person realizes are senseless but cannot control. Narcissistic personality disorder is marked by a pattern of self-involvement, grandiosity, and demand for constant attention.

## 19 Correct answer—**D**

A person with an antisocial personality typically is unable to form long-term emotional attachments. He usually has no friends and establishes relationships by manipulating others to satisfy his own needs. Indiscriminate sexual behavior with little concern for the other person's welfare is common. This type of egotistical behavior is most likely a defense against low self-esteem rather than a demonstration of high self-esteem and a strong self-concept. A patient with an antisocial personality tends to be relatively free of anxiety and does not experience remorse or guilt about his behavior. Although patients with antisocial personality tend to act out sexually, they usually do not exhibit sexual addiction. A person with a sexual addiction continues to be involved in sexual encounters that he realizes are harmful. Like many addicts, the sexually addicted person recognizes the consequences of his actions but cannot refrain from this behavior.

## 20 Correct answer—**B**

In responding to B., the nurse should be direct, clear, and non-rejecting. Telling B. that removing his shirt will provide the necessary access to his arm is an appropriate response. She should avoid commenting on his attractiveness and discourage rather than encourage B.'s seductive behavior. If the nurse feels that a male staff member is needed, she should state this clearly and decisively to demonstrate that she is in control of the situation. The nurse should avoid becoming further involved with B.'s provocative talk and should refocus on the need for him to remove his shirt for the blood pressure reading.

## 21 Correct answer—**B**

B.'s treatment should help him to recognize and observe limits while interacting with others. Achieving such a goal will be most difficult; it will require consistency on the part of the entire staff as they help the patient to develop effective coping skills to decrease his antisocial behavior and manipulation of others. The treatment plan should focus on helping B. to develop a sense of responsibility for his present behaviors rather than remorse over past misdeeds. After the patient has successfully developed coping skills for everyday relationships, he can begin focusing on career options and developing long-term, meaningful relationships with others.

## 22 Correct answer—D

Providing a structured environment and setting clear limits is essential for any patient who lacks self-discipline, has poor judgment, and manipulates others for his own gain. Caring for the patient yet ensuring that he adheres to certain restrictions can curb his maladaptive behaviors and eventually help him to develop self-control. Medications are of limited value in such patients unless they are needed to control severe aggressive outbursts. Confrontations over authority and limit setting should be handled matter-of-factly and limited to a brief restatement of the rules and consequences of noncompliance. The patient does not need to be restricted from other patients unless he fails to comply with the rules and takes advantage of others; then, he should be separated from other patients for only a specified period.

## 23 Correct answer—C

The best way for the nurse to respond to B.'s request to leave the unit when she is unaware of his privilege status is to state the facts about her vacation and the need to check his report. Even though the nurse is aware that B. may be trying to manipulate her, an honest, direct response helps build a trusting nurse-patient relationship and demonstrates respect. The nurse should not allow the patient to leave the unit before checking his status. This is especially true for patients with a history of manipulative behavior, such as those with antisocial personality. Belittling the patient and apologizing for having to check his status are inappropriate.

## 24 Correct answer—B

Confronting B. privately with the information is the best initial approach. It provides an opportunity for B. to respond while letting him know that staff members are aware of his alleged behavior. In a one-to-one session, the nurse can restate the limits regarding such behavior, further validate their occurrence, and stress their consequences. Not confronting B. and waiting until the reported behavior is confirmed would allow him to continue his actions and reinforce the notion that he can get away with unacceptable behavior. Also, by not acting on the other patients' concerns, the nurse risks being seen as nonsupportive of their feelings and concerns. Asking the patients involved to confront B. in a community meeting would probably be too threatening—B. may attempt to intimidate them while denying their claims about his behavior. Once the extent of B.'s manipulative behaviors is determined, the nurse can consider restricting or supervising his interactions with other patients.

## 25 Correct answer—C

The nurse must confront both patients about their behavior. She should explain why physical contact and other sexual behaviors are prohibited and clearly state the unit's rules regarding appropriate behavior. Waiting for further evidence of sexual behavior suggests to the patients that these actions are acceptable. Allowing the behavior to continue not only makes it more difficult to stop later but also places the female patient at risk for pregnancy should the encounters progress to intercourse. Counseling each patient about safe sex implies that such behaviors are permitted and condoned on the unit. Telling B. that he must end his relationship with the other patient is too harsh and does not allow him the opportunity to learn how to relate in a more mature manner.

## 26 Correct answer—D

Since the group leader has clearly stated the limits for B.'s behavior and has explained the consequences of noncompliance with the rules, she should tell B. in a matter-of-fact manner to leave the group. Setting limits is an important part of the treatment and must be done consistently. Ignoring B.'s comments would be an inappropriate response; the nurse should respond to the patient's refusal to cooperate directly and without delay. Asking the group to respond to B.'s work or his remarks probably will prolong the behavior rather than stop it.

## 27 Correct answer—A

Borderline personality disorder is characterized by a lack of self-esteem, strong dependency needs, and impulsive behavior. Instability in interpersonal relationships, mood, and self-image also is common. The patient typically cannot tolerate being alone, and she expresses feelings of emptiness or boredom. Flat affect, social withdrawal, and unusual dress are characteristic of schizoid personality disorder. Suspiciousness, hypervigilance, and emotional coldness are seen in patients with paranoid personality disorders. Patients with antisocial personality disorders usually are insensitive to others and act out sexually; they also may be violent.

## 28 Correct answer—A

By encouraging the patient to discuss how she feels, the nurse helps M. recognize her feelings of frustration and anger and explore them in a safe, therapeutic way. The focus should be on M. and her response, not the nurse's feelings about the incident. Although the nurse may want to apologize for being late, an apology is not enough; the nurse must also confront M.'s feelings of anger and rejection. Accusing M. of overreacting belittles her emotions and is nontherapeutic. Apologizing and arranging for reassignment does not help the patient express her feelings; learning to ventilate such feelings is especially important for a depressed patient.

## 29 Correct answer—C

Heroin is a short-acting drug. Early symptoms of withdrawal—usually seen within 8 to 12 hours after the last dose—include drug cravings, anxiety, yawning, increased perspiration, lacrimation, rhinorrhea, and sleeping problems. Later symptoms include irritability, dilated pupils, aching bones and muscles, piloerection, and hot and cold flashes. Withdrawal symptoms usually peak 48 to 72 hours after the last dose. If untreated, the withdrawal syndrome can last from 7 to 10 days.

## 30 Correct answer—D

The nurse should call the admitting physician or the physician in the detoxification unit to review the order. Methadone (Dolophine) doses of 10 to 20 mg every 2 hours as needed, but not to exceed 120 mg/day, usually are sufficient to control withdrawal symptoms. Only if the patient ingested pure heroin would higher doses be needed. The prescribed dosage—40 mg every 6 hours—is equivalent to a dosage of 160 mg/day, which is above the current federal guidelines of 120 mg/day and cannot be administered without special approval. Because the dosage ordered exceeds federal limits, the nurse should not administer the medication without first questioning the physician. Dissolving the dose in juice is an appropriate method of administering methadone, but only after the nurse clarifies the order. Asking the patient about his drug history is irrelevant to the situation.

## 31 Correct answer—**D**

Heroin abusers who inject themselves are at high risk for acquired immunodeficiency syndrome (AIDS). Addicts frequently share needles and other drug paraphernalia with little regard for sterility. The incidence of AIDS among the drug-abusing population is a serious problem. Addicts also are at risk for such infections as endocarditis, septicemia, tuberculosis, and syphilis because of poor hygiene, indiscriminant and unprotected sex, poor nutrition, and shared needles. The nurse must observe universal precautions for blood and other body fluids when treating drug abusers to protect herself and other patients. These precautions include properly disposing of needles and wearing gloves when drawing blood, changing dressings, or coming in contact with body fluids.

## 32 Correct answer—**A**

Therapeutic communities are long-term treatment programs, generally requiring a commitment of 12 to 18 months in residence. Various programs are available, including some run primarily by former addicts and some by professional staff and ex-addicts. These programs attempt to help the addict change his life-style, abstain from drug use, and develop new coping skills. These drug-free environments do not permit methadone or other drug substitutes as part of the treatment. Outpatient day treatment programs attempt to foster similar goals within a therapeutic community setting for an addict who cannot commit to long-term residential treatment.

# CHAPTER 8

# Chronic
# or Terminal
# Illness

## Questions

**1** When caring for a dying patient, the nurse should give priority to:

**A.** Managing the patient's physical symptoms
**B.** Increasing the patient's decision-making opportunities
**C.** Facilitating the patient's expression of feelings
**D.** Involving the patient's family in his care

**2** Which communication technique is most important when working with a dying patient and his family?

**A.** Reflection
**B.** Interpretation
**C.** Clarification
**D.** Active listening

**3** The nurse is sitting with a patient who is crying over having had a breast removed because of cancer. The nurse becomes uncomfortable after the crying continues for 5 minutes. The nurse should:

**A.** Encourage the patient to talk about another topic
**B.** Attempt to comfort the patient by putting an arm around her
**C.** Continue to sit in silence
**D.** Leave the room and tell the patient that she will return

**4** Denial is a common initial response to serious illness, amputation, and impending death. The nurse's response to a patient's denial should be:

**A.** Confrontational
**B.** Accepting
**C.** Supportive
**D.** Interpretive

### SITUATION

*P.K., age 52, is diagnosed with metastatic cancer and has less than 6 months to live. He is being cared for at home by his wife and four children with the support of a home health care nurse who visits twice a week. P. is a proud, uncomplaining man who has not yet talked about his illness or approaching death with anyone.*

*Questions 5 to 8 refer to this situation.*

**5** The nurse knows that a dying patient should be encouraged to talk about death and dying. The most therapeutic approach is to:

**A.** Confront P. with the facts about his illness and impending death to prompt an open discussion
**B.** Encourage family members to raise the issue of dying
**C.** Verify that the physician has told P. about his diagnosis and prognosis before initiating a discussion
**D.** Remain available and listen carefully for cues that P. is ready to discuss his impending death

**6** P. begins deteriorating markedly. He requires frequent pain medication and is confused when conscious. His oldest daughter, J., age 21, walks out of his room crying and says to the nurse, "I wish he would just die. I can't take this any more." How should the nurse respond?

**A.** "It is difficult to see someone you love suffer. Let's go outside and talk about how you're feeling"
**B.** "He probably will die soon. He's getting weaker every day"
**C.** "I hope your father didn't hear you. He needs all the support you can give him right now"
**D.** "You say that you can't take it any more. Can you imagine how this struggle has been for him?"

**7** Mrs. K. tells the nurse that during a lucid period, her husband was able to talk about his dying. She says that he did not appear frightened and seemed at peace with himself, saying that he loved his family and would miss them very much but that he felt his time had come. Mrs. K. asks the nurse if her husband has given up the will to live. The nurse should reply:

**A.** "I really can't answer that question. No one knows when it is their turn to die"
**B.** "You said he seemed at peace, rather than hopeless. Could it be that he's accepting his dying?"
**C.** "Do you think he has resigned himself to the fact that he is dying?"
**D.** "Have you given up on him?"

**8** Six months after her husband dies, Mrs. K. calls the home health care nurse. She reports that she still cries when she thinks about her husband and their life together and that her children seem to have handled their father's death better than she has. Which response is most helpful?

**A.** "Each person grieves in his own way. It can take a year or more for you to recover from the loss of your husband"
**B.** "You have to give yourself time. Six months is not very long. Of course you're still sad"
**C.** "Why don't you ask your children how they've been handling their feelings?"
**D.** "Perhaps if you remain busy, you'll be able to keep your mind on other things"

---

## SITUATION

*C.R., age 41, is scheduled to undergo a breast biopsy after a mammography offered by a local women's clinic revealed a small lump in her breast. She completes her preadmission testing early in the morning and is admitted at 7:30 a.m. the same day.*

*Questions 9 to 13 refer to this situation.*

---

**9** The admitting nurse reviews preoperative and postoperative procedures with C. When the nurse asks if she has any questions, C. replies, "I wish I had never gone for that mammography." How should the nurse respond?

**A.** "Don't say that, C. Early detection through mammography is the key to effective treatment"
**B.** "Why do you say that, C.?"
**C.** "Don't be afraid. Most breast lumps are benign. It's better to be safe than sorry"
**D.** "C., what are you thinking and feeling right now?"

**10** As the nurse prepares to administer the preoperative medications, C. begins to cry and says that she knows her husband will be repulsed by her if her "breast is cut off and she has a big ugly scar." Which response is most therapeutic at this time?

**A.** "If a mastectomy is necessary, there will be a period of adjustment for both you and your husband. We can help you through that"
**B.** "Sometimes the scars are not as bad as you expect. Why not wait and see what happens during the biopsy?"
**C.** "This medication should help you relax. We can talk after your biopsy"
**D.** "It's best not to cross that bridge until you come to it. Right now you're only going for a biopsy"

**11** C.'s biopsy is positive for cancer. Her physician discusses the available treatment options and recommends a total mastectomy. C. says to the nurse, "The physician said I could have a lumpectomy and radiation, but he recommends total removal of my breast. What do you think I should do?" Which response is most appropriate?

**A.** "I really can't give my opinion on that. It's between you and your physician"
**B.** "You have a difficult decision to make. What does your husband want you to do?"
**C.** "You may want to consider getting a second opinion before making your decision"
**D.** "If I were you, I think I'd choose the least disfiguring operation"

**12** C. decides to undergo a total mastectomy. Mr. R. asks the nurse how he can help his wife cope with the loss of her breast. Which suggestion is most helpful?

**A.** "Just be there for her. That's most important"
**B.** "She needs to know you love her and are not afraid to talk about how you both feel about the mastectomy"
**C.** "Be sure she knows you love her with or without her breast"
**D.** "Try to keep her spirits up. Avoid talking about cancer and the mastectomy until she is stronger"

**13** C. is reluctant to exercise her affected arm because it is too painful. The nurse can encourage her to exercise by:

**A.** Arranging for another woman who has undergone a successful mastectomy for breast cancer to speak with her
**B.** Explaining that if she does not exercise, she will lose mobility in her arm
**C.** Having the physician talk with her about the importance of exercise
**D.** Recognizing that she is grieving over her lost breast and will resume exercising once she has resolved her grief

## SITUATION

*J., a 29-year-old homosexual male, is diagnosed as having acquired immunodeficiency syndrome (AIDS). He currently is hospitalized on the medical unit for treatment of* Pneumocystis carinii pneumonia. *His lover and a few friends visit him in the hospital. J. states that his family does not know he is homosexual or that he has AIDS.*

*Questions 14 to 18 refer to this situation.*

**14** One afternoon J. says to the nurse, "Do you think God is punishing me for being homosexual?" Which response is most therapeutic?

**A.** "I really can't say. Some people do think AIDS is a punishment for homosexuality"
**B.** "I think it would be best if you discussed this with the hospital chaplain. Should I call him for you?"
**C.** "AIDS is an illness. Are you saying you feel like you're being punished?"
**D.** "Do you think God is punishing you?"

**15** Several of J.'s friends have been encouraging him to inform his family of his illness. He tells the nurse that he is afraid his family would reject him completely and that he would then be really alone. The best way to explore his feelings is to say:

**A.** "I don't think you're giving your parents enough credit. You are their son. I'm sure they love you very much"
**B.** "You need to make up your mind for yourself. Don't let your friends pressure you into doing something you are uncomfortable with"
**C.** "You are quite ill. Let's talk about your fears and how telling your family could be a source of support or a problem for you"
**D.** "Families are very important when one is ill. Why don't you give them a chance?"

**16** The nurse overhears a nursing assistant remark, "He's really disgusting. He's in there holding hands with another man. Don't they know that AIDS is spread by sexual contact?" The nurse talks with the assistant privately about her remark. The nurse can help most by saying:

**A.** "You really shouldn't be so judgmental about J.'s behavior. He's a human being with human needs"
**B.** "I'd like to discuss your remarks about J. and his visitor. I'm particularly concerned about your calling him 'disgusting'"
**C.** "You know that AIDS is not spread by casual contact, such as holding hands, so why did you call him disgusting?"
**D.** "I don't want to hear you make any more remarks in public about the patients here. It's unethical"

**17** The nursing assistant tells the nurse that, according to her religious beliefs, homosexuality is a sin and that she cannot help feeling repulsed by J.'s behavior. How should the nurse reply?

**A.** "I understand how important your religion is to you and why you feel this way. I apologize for criticizing you"
**B.** "I appreciate your right to believe as you do, but you must put your beliefs aside and take care of your patient"
**C.** "Do you think that judging J. by your religious beliefs is fair to him?"
**D.** "It is difficult to put such deeply held beliefs aside. Let's talk about J.'s need for comfort and support"

**18** J. decides to contact his parents. When his mother visits, he tells her that he is homosexual and has AIDS. As his mother leaves the room, she meets the nurse. She is crying and says, "How could I know so little about my own son? Now it's too late to get to know him." The nurse can be most supportive by responding:

**A.** "Don't punish yourself. Your son didn't let you know him until now"

**B.** "It's not too late. Your son should recuperate from this hospitalization"

**C.** "It is sad when family members are estranged from one another. I understand how you must be feeling"

**D.** "You are here now for him and you can begin to learn about each other"

---

## SITUATION

*R.W., age 18, is brought to the emergency department after suffering extensive brain and internal injuries in an automobile accident. Her prognosis is poor. Her parents arrive at the hospital after being notified by the police; they are extremely distraught. R. is their only child, and they demand to see her immediately, despite being informed that the trauma team is treating her.*

*Questions 19 to 21 refer to this situation.*

---

**19** Mr. and Mrs. W. beg the nurse to let them see R. "just for a minute, so we know she's all right." How should the nurse respond?

**A.** "I realize you are worried about your daughter, but we're doing all we can to help her right now. I'll call you if there is any change"

**B.** "I don't think you want to see R. right now. The trauma team is working on her, and it's not a pretty sight. Please wait outside until you are called"

**C.** "I understand your concern about R. The trauma team is treating her right now, and they are busy and the room is small. I'll keep you informed and bring you in as soon as possible"

**D.** "Hospital rules prohibit families from being in the room during treatment of such severe trauma. I promise to bring you in to see R. as soon as possible"

**20** R. dies despite the trauma team's efforts. Her parents are informed in a private area and request to see their daughter's body. Mrs. W. looks at R.'s body and screams, "Oh my God, that's not my daughter. It can't be. Not my baby girl." Which response is most therapeutic at this time?

**A.** Saying gently, "Mrs. W., this is R. We have identified her. I'm sorry, there is no mistake"
**B.** Saying, "I know this is difficult for you to accept," then asking Mr. W. to escort his wife from the room and comfort her
**C.** Saying nothing while standing by Mr. and Mrs. W. and allowing them to express their grief
**D.** Explaining to Mrs. W. that R. may look different because of the accident and treatment, but that it is her daughter

**21** The nurse realizes that Mr. and Mrs. W.'s ability to cope with the sudden death of their daughter will probably require:

**A.** Consistent support systems
**B.** Psychotherapy
**C.** Six months of grieving
**D.** Use of tricyclic antidepressants

## SITUATION

*A., age 16, is a patient on the medical unit. Diagnostic testing confirms that she has insulin-dependent diabetes mellitus.*

*Questions 22 to 26 refer to this situation.*

**22** After the diagnosis is explained to her, A. appears to accept it and asks many questions about diabetes and its management. The nurse anticipates that A.:

**A.** Has made a positive adjustment to her disease
**B.** Will be easy to work with because of her accepting attitude
**C.** May still experience anger and denial of her illness
**D.** Is not yet coping with her illness

**23** After the nurse reviews the diabetic exchange list, A. remarks, "I'll never have any friends now. After school we all go to a fast food restaurant and hang out. What am I supposed to do—eat an apple?" Which is the best reponse?

**A.** "You have a serious disease. Proper diet is the most important factor in staying healthy"
**B.** "You'll have to make some changes in your eating habits. Let's see how we can plan for those afternoons"
**C.** "Fast foods are the worst. They're high in calories and cholesterol. You'd be better off with that apple"
**D.** "Are you really concerned about what your friends will think?"

**24** The nurse has several meetings with A. regarding insulin, diet, rest, exercise, and daily schedule. A. comments, "Do I have to lead the rest of my life around a clock?" The most helpful response would be:

**A.** "It's not as bad as it sounds. You can lead a normal life"
**B.** "In many ways you do. How do you feel about that?"
**C.** "Is that really so bad?"
**D.** "If you want to be healthy, you have to plan your day. Can you live with that?"

**25** The nurse plans to teach A. relaxation techniques to control stress. These techniques are especially important for patients such as A. because:

**A.** Stress is usually handled inappropriately by teenagers
**B.** Stress produces symptoms similar to those of insulin shock
**C.** Proper rest is important for patients with diabetes
**D.** Biofeedback is usually ineffective with teenagers

**26** Which of the following will be most beneficial to A. in helping her adjust to her diabetes?

**A.** Peer support group
**B.** Nutritional counseling
**C.** Psychotherapy
**D.** Visiting nurse

## Answer sheet

```
    A B C D
 1 ○○○○
 2 ○○○○
 3 ○○○○
 4 ○○○○
 5 ○○○○
 6 ○○○○
 7 ○○○○
 8 ○○○○
 9 ○○○○
10 ○○○○
11 ○○○○
12 ○○○○
13 ○○○○
14 ○○○○
15 ○○○○
16 ○○○○
17 ○○○○
18 ○○○○
19 ○○○○
20 ○○○○
21 ○○○○
22 ○○○○
23 ○○○○
24 ○○○○
25 ○○○○
26 ○○○○
```

# Answers and rationales

## 1 Correct answer—A

Managing the patient's physical symptoms—relieving pain and tending to hygiene, respiration, elimination, comfort, and other physical needs that the patient cannot meet himself—should be the nurse's priority when caring for a dying patient. Meeting physical needs reassures the patient and his family about the adequacy of the care being provided. After meeting the patient's physical needs, the nurse can attempt to increase decision-making opportunities, such as allowing the patient to decide the time for his bath. Facilitating the patient's expression of feelings and involving family members in the patient's care also are important but are not the priority at this time.

## 2 Correct answer—D

Active listening—empathically responding to another person's feelings while remaining aware of one's own feelings—is the most important communication skill the nurse can use when working with the dying patient and his family. This communication technique allows the nurse to assess the patient's and family's feelings and coping skills and to determine their immediate and long-term needs. It also enables the nurse to select other appropriate communication strategies, such as silence, reflection (repeating essential ideas), and clarification (putting implied thoughts into words), when interacting with the patient and family members. Interpretation—drawing inferences about the patient's behaviors and then confronting the patient—should be used sparingly and at the proper time to avoid placing the patient on the defensive.

## 3 Correct answer—D

When a nurse cannot control her own feelings of discomfort in front of the patient, she should temporarily leave the room to examine her emotions and reactions. A nurse who becomes extremely uncomfortable or anxious while interacting with a patient may inadvertently communicate uninterest or disapproval. If the nurse cannot resolve her discomfort, she should ask another nurse to talk with the patient. Because the therapeutic goal is to facilitate and support the patient through her grieving, changing the topic would not be helpful. Attempting to console the patient by putting an arm around her is appropriate only if both the nurse and patient are comfortable with this approach. If the nurse continues to sit in

silence without addressing her uneasiness, she may unintention-
ally convey her own discomfort to the patient.

---

**4** Correct answer—**B**

Whenever a patient is faced with serious illness, body image alterations (such as amputation), or imminent death, the nurse should
respond by helping the patient to cope with change. One way to
accomplish this is by allowing the patient to express his feelings,
including anger and depression. By accepting the patient's initial
denial, the nurse acknowledges the role that denial plays in the
coping process. Interpreting the patient's denial (drawing inferences about his behavior) and then confronting him will increase
his anxiety, hinder development of a trusting relationship, and
delay the patient's acceptance of his condition. Accepting the
patient's expression of denial does not imply that the nurse supports his denial.

---

**5** Correct answer—**D**

Because each patient deals with dying individually, the nurse
should remain available and listen carefully for cues from the patient that he is ready to discuss dying. Trying to force the patient
to discuss his feelings or to confront him before he is ready is an
unproductive strategy that may discourage the patient from attempting any further communication. The nurse should encourage
the family members to be available and to listen for similar cues
that the patient is ready to talk, but they should not be asked to initiate a discussion about dying. Although the nurse should confirm
what the physician and family members have told the patient
about his illness, she should remain alert to the possibility that the
patient may wish to verbalize his concerns at any time, even before he learns that he is dying. Asking a patient how he feels is
often a good way to encourage verbalization of fears. The patient
may want or need to discuss what is happening to him regardless
of what the physician has or has not told him; the nurse should be
available to the patient for these discussions.

---

**6** Correct answer—**A**

One of the nurse's responsibilities in this situation is to offer support and facilitate the family's grieving. The nurse can best help J.
by empathically reflecting the difficulty she is experiencing seeing
her father suffer and by offering her an opportunity to ventilate
her feelings. Telling J. that her father will be dead soon does not

address the real issue—J.'s difficulty with seeing her father suffer. Saying "I hope your father didn't hear you" or "Can you imagine how this struggle has been for him?" are insensitive and judgmental responses that would only add to J.'s stress and grief by making her feel guilty about her emotions.

## 7 Correct answer—**B**

By restating that Mrs. K. described her husband as at peace rather than hopeless, the nurse tries to help her understand that P. may be accepting his death. As outlined by Kübler-Ross, acceptance is the final stage of grieving (the earlier stages are shock and denial, anger and rage, bargaining, and depression). During the final stage, the dying person begins to disengage from those around him. By helping Mrs. K. understand the dying process, the nurse can help her meet her husband's needs and prepare herself for his death. Telling Mrs. K. that no one knows when they will die or asking her if she has given up on her husband does not encourage her to develop an understanding of the dying process. Asking whether she thinks her husband is resigned to the fact that he is dying conveys that giving up (resignation) is a normal part of the grieving process. The nurse should help Mrs. K. to realize that her husband's behavior suggests he finally has accepted his impending death.

## 8 Correct answer—**A**

Mrs. K. is asking for reassurance that her grieving is normal. Informing her that grief is an individualized response and that recovering from the loss of a spouse can take a year or more provides support and reassurance. This approach is better than telling her to give herself time, which might be interpreted as a nonaccepting and judgmental response. The loss of a spouse is an experience different from that of the loss of a parent. Although communication within the family is important, the nurse—not Mrs. K.'s children—must respond to her request for help. Advising Mrs. K. only to keep busy implies that her grieving is unacceptable.

## 9 Correct answer—**D**

The nurse should encourage the patient to discuss her fears and concerns. The nurse can facilitate this process by asking the patient directly what she is thinking and feeling. After eliciting the patient's fears and concerns, the nurse should offer support by presenting the facts about the biopsy and its possible outcomes. Although it is true that 8 of 10 biopsies reveal nonmalignant tissue, comments such as "Don't say that" or "Don't be afraid" deny the validity of the patient's concerns and may sound like false reassurance. "Why" questions can be difficult for the patient to answer and should generally be avoided.

## 10 Correct answer—A

By recognizing the patient's concerns about her body image and her husband's response to mastectomy, the nurse can offer honest reassurance about what will happen after the procedure. If a mastectomy is necessary, the patient and her husband can expect a period of grieving; staff members will be available to help both of them through it. An honest, caring response is more helpful than attempts to deny, ignore, or put off the patient's concerns.

## 11 Correct answer—C

The nurse's role is to assist the patient in the decision-making process. Because C. is expressing a need for more information about available treatment options, the nurse can help by suggesting that she seek a second opinion. The nurse should provide professional advice and direction and not ignore the patient's needs. Although the patient probably will discuss her decision with her husband, his opinion is secondary to the patient's at this time. It would be inappropriate for the nurse to respond by giving an opinion based on her personal needs.

## 12 Correct answer—B

Mr. R.'s participation in his wife's recovery is crucial and should be encouraged and supported. He can best help his wife adjust to the loss of her breast by both expressing his love and being willing to talk about the mastectomy with her. Most difficulties in these situations are caused by a lack of communication between spouses, which leads to feelings of fear, rejection, and negative body image. The nurse's response should facilitate communication between the patient and her husband. A husband who actively participates in his wife's care can have the greatest effect during recovery of a mastectomy. Just "being there" or expressing love is not enough. The nurse should encourage Mr. R. to discuss the cancer as well as the mastectomy with his wife so that they may explore their feelings and thoughts about how the cancer and surgery have affected their lives.

**13** Correct answer—A

Because most patients receive a high degree of encouragement and motivation from someone who has successfully undergone the same type of surgery or been in a similar situation, the nurse should contact the local American Cancer Society or Reach to Recovery to have a volunteer speak with C. In many cases, a patient who has had a mastectomy will listen more readily to the advice of a woman who has experienced similar problems and feelings than she would to a nurse or a physician. It may be true that without exercise, C.'s shoulder may become immobile in as little as 4 to 5 days and that lymphatic drainage is promoted by exercise; however, telling C. that if she does not exercise, she will lose mobility is a confrontational and threatening response. The patient's grieving over the loss of her breast may continue for several months; exercise cannot be delayed for that long.

**14** Correct answer—C

The nurse must demonstrate acceptance of the patient and clearly state that acquired immunodeficiency syndrome (AIDS) is an illness. She then can explore any feelings the patient may have about being punished for his life-style. Refusing to take a position and merely restating that some people think AIDS is a punishment is a judgmental, nonsupportive response. The patient is asking the nurse for feedback—referring him to the chaplain would appear as if she were avoiding or distancing herself from the patient. Reflecting the patient's question back to him may stimulate discussion, but it is a nontherapeutic approach because it focuses on the issue of punishment and not the reality that AIDS is a disease.

**15** Correct answer—C

The nurse should help the patient express his feelings about his family while focusing on the reality of his condition. Instead of voicing her opinion about what J. should or should not do, the nurse should encourage him to discuss the pros and cons of telling his family about his situation. The patient's decision to contact his family should not be based on peer pressure or the nurse's biases, values, or attitudes about families, homosexuality, or AIDS.

## 16 Correct answer—B

One role of the professional nurse is to facilitate expression of feelings and fears by staff members working with AIDS patients. In this situation, the nurse should use an assertive, confrontational tone and tell the nursing assistant that she wants to discuss her remarks about the patient and his visitor. She also should express concern about the assistant's calling the patient disgusting. This approach sets the stage for exploring the aide's fears, beliefs, and attitudes without condemning or lecturing her. During the ensuing discussion, the nurse can clarify and restate information about the importance of support and comfort from others during illness, how AIDS is transmitted, and the role of hospital personnel in meeting patient needs.

## 17 Correct answer—D

In responding to the nursing assistant's comments about her religion, the nurse must realize that such deeply held beliefs are not easily changed. The nurse can be most helpful by acknowledging the conflict that the assistant is experiencing and then working with her to identify J.'s needs for emotional comfort and support. Approaching the problem this way meets the needs of both the patient and the aide. Recognizing the assistant's beliefs and apologizing to her does not provide a way to meet J.'s needs. Expecting the assistant to set aside her beliefs is unrealistic; telling her to do so would be inappropriate and result in a missed opportunity to teach her how to confront her feelings for J. in an appropriate manner. Responding in a judgmental manner would elicit a defensive response from the assistant and shift the focus of the discussion away from the needs of the patient.

## 18 Correct answer—D

The nurse can help J.'s mother by telling her, in a supportive and positive way, that she and her son can use whatever time is left to learn about each other. Consistent, honest, and open communication is important when working with an AIDS patient and his family members. False reassurances, such as "It's not too late," and nonempathic advice, such as "Don't punish yourself," are inappropriate. Focusing on past estrangement may induce more guilt and interfere with the mother's ability to get to know her son better.

**19** Correct answer—**C**

The nurse should respond to R.'s parents with empathic assertiveness. This is accomplished by recognizing their concerns, explaining why they cannot see their daughter, and reassuring them that they will be kept informed and brought in as soon as possible. Recognizing that they are worried and stating "We're doing all we can" does not help the parents understand what to expect next. They are unlikely to be reassured by the nurse's insensitive comment, "It's not a pretty sight." Reciting hospital rules distances the nurse from the parents with its formality.

**20** Correct answer—**C**

The nurse should demonstrate her understanding of the grieving process by accepting the parents' reaction of shock and denial and remaining with them at this time. The death of a child is a severe psychological trauma for the parents, and the unexpectedness of the death compounds the impact. The parents need time to cope with the event, and the nurse can be more supportive with her quiet presence than by trying to convince them that this is their daughter's body.

**21** Correct answer—**A**

Coping with the sudden death of a child, particularly an only child, produces severe stress for the parents. Successful coping depends on the parent's ability to identify and use consistent support systems as they try to deal with their loss. Some parents may seek professional assistance, such as psychotherapy, when support systems are inadequate or absent. Grieving is unique to each person; the time required varies but typically lasts a year or longer. Antidepressants usually are unnecessary; many parents in this situation feel the need to grieve and overcome their depression by working through the grieving process.

**22** Correct answer—**C**

The nurse should anticipate that A. may still experience a period of anger and even denial concerning her diabetes. Type I (insulin-dependent) diabetes is a lifelong illness that is difficult to accept at any age, possibly more so during the teenage years. The nurse must provide support and understanding to help the patient work through her anger and denial and develop a sense of control over her life. It would be premature to assume that A. has made a positive adjustment to her illness or that she is not yet coping with it. Even though the patient initially appears to accept her condition, she may become less accepting once she moves into the anger and denial phase of coping.

## 23 Correct answer—B

The nurse can be most helpful by recognizing the importance of a teenager's peer-related activities and helping A. to find ways to plan her diet with these activities in mind. By reinforcing that changes in her eating habits are necessary and by agreeing to work with her, the nurse can help the patient identify positive habits and coping strategies. Lecturing A. about the seriousness of her disease or the nutritional value of fast foods is a nonempathic response that does not encourage her to explore ways of modifying her life-style. The nurse must keep in mind that peer acceptance is critical to a teenager's self-esteem; asking A. whether she is really concerned about what her friends think would be inappropriate.

## 24 Correct answer—B

The reality of A.'s question must be addressed. A diabetic patient must plan for meals, insulin, exercise, and rest and to a great extent must live by the clock. The nurse's answer acknowledges this reality and seeks to explore A.'s feelings about it. At age 16, A. is trying to become more independent and may resent the rules and regulations her illness places on her. Although she cannot lead a "normal" life, she can lead a healthy one with proper management. By creating an atmosphere of empathy and acceptance, the nurse can facilitate the patient's expression of feelings. Responses such as "It's not as bad as it sounds," "Is that really so bad?" or "Can you live with that?" devalue the patient's feelings.

## 25 Correct answer—B

The symptoms of stress—irritability, sweating, mood changes, crying, shaking, and headache—resemble those of insulin shock. Stress can mask the onset of insulin shock, possibly delaying appropriate treatment. Stress also can lead to metabolic decompensation, further interfering with diabetes management. The teenage years are a time of great stress, but with support from family and friends, teenagers usually handle stress quite well. Diabetic patients need adequate rest, but rest does not reduce stress. Biofeedback is a relaxation technique that enables a patient to develop an awareness of how stress affects the body; it can be taught to any motivated individual, including a teenager.

## 26 Correct answer—A

A peer support group, composed of other teenage diabetic patients, can provide the encouragement A. needs at this time. Teenagers usually respond best to other teenagers and are more likely to accept advice from each other than from an adult. Teenage support groups typically include a health team member who is available to clarify diet, medication, and other management issues. Nutritional counseling, psychotherapy, and visiting nurse services will be appropriate if A. requires additional professional support to help her adapt to her condition.

# CHAPTER 9

# Childhood and Adolescent Disorders

## Questions

**1** Behavior problems in children are most commonly a sign of:

A. Inability to cope with stress
B. Autistic thinking
C. Loss of contact with reality
D. Psychosis

**2** When caring for a child with Tourette's syndrome, the nurse finds that the physician has prescribed methylphenidate (Ritalin) 1 mg b.i.d. Which nursing action would be most appropriate at this time?

A. Administer the medication as ordered
B. Assess the patient for weight gain
C. Question the medication order
D. Check the patient's pulse before giving the medication

**3** The school nurse is caring for L., a 16-year-old girl who has been seen vomiting in the lavatory after lunch on several occasions during the past few months. L. tells the nurse that she had a fight with her boyfriend earlier in the day, then consumed two pizzas, 1 gallon of ice cream, and 2 liters of soda at lunch in order to make herself vomit. The nurse realizes that this type of behavior is characteristic of someone with:

A. Bulimia
B. Conduct disorder
C. Anorexia nervosa
D. Gluttony

**4** Psychologically, a bulimic patient differs from an anorexic patient through awareness that her behavior is:

A. Acceptable for maintaining weight
B. Abnormal
C. Easy to control
D. Physically dangerous

**5** The personality of a bulimic patient differs from·that of an anorexic patient in that she is commonly:

A. Impulsive
B. Controlled
C. Serious
D. Intelligent

## SITUATION

*L., a 12-year-old girl, is admitted to the psychiatric unit for severe anxiety. The admitting nurse notices that the child appears frightened. L. tells the nurse that she has "never been in a place like this before." Her history reveals that she has been hearing voices for the past several days.*

*Questions 6 to 8 refer to this situation.*

**6** Which question or statement by the nurse would be inappropriate during the initial patient interview?

**A.** "Have you recently used any drugs?"
**B.** "Tell me what the voice you heard said to you"
**C.** "You are not really hearing voices. You just think you do"
**D.** "Have you heard these voices before?"

**7** The day after her admission, L. points to an empty chair and says, "Don't sit on Daddy." How should the nurse reply?

**A.** "L., you know that Daddy isn't in that chair"
**B.** "All right, I'll sit in another chair"
**C.** "I see no one in the room besides you and me"
**D.** "Would Daddy like to go to the recreation hall with us?"

**8** Several days later, L. begins to follow the nurse around and talk quietly with her. Which approach would best help L. relate to others?

**A.** Ask the most outgoing patient on the unit to talk with L.
**B.** Leave L. with a large group of patients
**C.** Invite a calm, sensitive patient to join L. and the nurse in a conversation
**D.** Allow L. to decide for herself whether to interact with the other patients

## SITUATION

*T., age 2, is accompanied to the pediatric clinic by his parents, who report that he frequently bangs his head, seems "slow," cries frequently, and is obsessively attached to his blanket. The nurse notes that T. demonstrates no evidence of babbling or speech, plays alone for hours with his teddy bear, and periodically makes bizarre arm movements.*

*Questions 9 to 12 refer to this situation.*

**9** Based on her initial observations, the nurse suspects that T. has a medical diagnosis of:

A. Early infantile autism
B. Moderate mental retardation
C. Antisocial personality
D. Paranoid personality

**10** Which approach is best for the nurse to take with T.?

A. Hold and cuddle him to make him feel secure
B. Ask his mother to temporarily give up care of him
C. Provide a safe, neutral environment for him
D. Have him admitted to the psychiatric unit

**11** The treatment of choice for T. probably will include:

A. Psychoanalysis
B. Behavior modification
C. Group therapy
D. Play therapy

**12** Primary treatment goals for T.'s recovery should include all of the following *except:*

A. Developing self-concept
B. Accepting healthy nurturance
C. Maintaining contact with reality
D. Encouraging T. to play with a ball

## SITUATION

*D., age 10, is admitted to the psychiatric unit by court order. His history reveals multiple delinquent acts, the most recent being arson at a local high school.*

*Questions 13 to 17 refer to this situation.*

**13** The nurse notes that D. is charming and witty but incapable of seeing anything wrong with what he does. This behavior is characteristic of:

A. Pervasive developmental disorder
B. Mental retardation
C. Antisocial conduct disorder
D. Separation anxiety disorder

**14** During the patient interview, D. elaborates on his history by telling stories. The nurse realizes that these stories are untrue and that they are:

A. Symptomatic of the diagnosis
B. D.'s way of belittling the nurse
C. Part of D.'s delusions
D. D.'s way of asking for help

**15** D. becomes increasingly manipulative during his stay on the unit. During a staff meeting, the nurses discuss ways to manage D.'s behavior better. Which statement best demonstrates an understanding of how to manage such antisocial behavior?

A. "D. needs our acceptance when he breaks the rules"
B. "D. will become more cooperative once he knows he will be discharged for this behavior"
C. "D. requires a more controlled environment and a consistent approach by all staff members"
D. "D. has guilt feelings that must be explored"

**16** Patients with antisocial (conduct) disorder typically have impaired functioning in all of the following areas *except:*

A. Emotional response
B. Social conscience
C. Judgment
D. Intellect

**17** The nursing team decides to try behavior modification with D. Which nursing action is most important when implementing this type of treatment?

**A.** Acquiring a medical history about the patient's previous hospitalizations
**B.** Establishing realistic patient goals
**C.** Confirming that all staff members agree on the treatment plan
**D.** Ensuring that the designated rewards are important to D.

---

### SITUATION

---

*R., a 6-year-old first grader, is referred to the community mental health clinic by the school nurse because of his continued disruptive behavior. The school nurse reports that R. does not pay attention in class, seems unable to remain in his seat for more than brief periods, ignores the teacher's directions, and frequently disrupts other children's activities. His behavior in kindergarten was reportedly the same.*

*Questions 18 and 19 refer to this situation.*

**18** R.'s mother believes that he is "just bored with the school environment because he is so bright." She asks the clinic nurse if she should transfer R. to a school in which he would receive more stimulation. How should the nurse reply?

**A.** "How do you think changing schools will help R.'s behavior?"
**B.** "It sounds to me like R. would find it difficult to make such a change"
**C.** "Tell me how R. behaves at home with you and your other children"
**D.** "I don't think it's wise to make such a decision until the evaluation is completed"

**19** R.'s parents and older brothers are asked to participate in interviews as part of R.'s diagnostic workup. The primary purpose of these interviews is to:

**A.** Assess family dynamics and identify each family member's perception of the problem
**B.** Assess family dynamics and provide family therapy as needed
**C.** Identify disorders or disruptions within the family system
**D.** Discuss how the family members can help R. to control his behavior

## SITUATION

*K., age 16, is brought to the adolescent clinic by her mother, who is worried that her daughter is becoming seriously ill. K. is 5′ (152 cm) tall and weighs 75 lb (34 kg). She consumes only 100 to 200 calories a day, appears emaciated, and has amenorrhea.*

*Questions 20 to 23 refer to this situation.*

**20** Which disorder should the nurse suspect based on the above history findings?

**A.** Bulimia
**B.** Pica
**C.** Compulsive eating disorder
**D.** Anorexia nervosa

**21** Which nursing diagnostic category is least applicable to this patient?

**A.** Ineffective individual coping
**B.** Body image disturbance
**C.** Altered nutrition, less than body requirements
**D.** Dressing and grooming self-care deficit

**22** Which nursing action is inappropriate for K. at this time?

**A.** Starting K. on a behavior modification program
**B.** Taking necessary measures to control K.'s manipulative behavior
**C.** Referring K. for psychotherapy
**D.** Using logic and reasoning to persuade K. to alter her behavior

**23** The nurse realizes that K.'s behavior probably is a result of her effort to:

**A.** Meet others' expectations
**B.** Live up to standard weight and height charts
**C.** Gain control over at least one aspect of her life
**D.** Satisfy peer pressure

## SITUATION

*B., an 18-year-old high school senior, went steady with his girlfriend for 1 year but broke up 2 months ago. Since then, he has exhibited sadness, fatigue, and poor concentration. He left his after-school job, failed two biology exams, and quit the basketball team. He was referred to the mental health center by the school counselor, who was concerned about B.'s behavior.*

*Questions 24 to 27 refer to this situation.*

**24** The nurse assesses B.'s behavior and suspects that it is probably:

**A.** A normal reaction to breaking up with his girlfriend
**B.** A result of ineffective coping related to depression
**C.** A consequence of fear of failing
**D.** An inconsequential problem and nothing to worry about

**25** While conducting the initial assessment, the nurse learns that B. drinks a six-pack of beer each night and has started smoking marijuana in his room. These actions are indicative of:

**A.** Normal teenage experimentation
**B.** Psychotic behavior disorder
**C.** Indirect self-destructive behavior
**D.** Direct self-destructive behavior

**26** When B. returns to the mental health center for his next visit, the nurse learns that he has stopped going to school and refuses to bathe or change his clothes. He tells the nurse that he consumed a fifth of whiskey and smoked two marijuana cigarettes before driving himself to the center at a speed of 75 mph. The nurse realizes that this type of behavior is considered:

**A.** Suicidal
**B.** Anxious
**C.** Depressed
**D.** Psychotic

**27** The physician calls for an immediate family conference to discuss B.'s problems and possible treatments. During the ensuing discussion, B.'s parents express extreme concern about his welfare and safety. When interacting with B. and his parents, the nurse should:

**A.** Side with B.'s parents
**B.** Side only with B.
**C.** Serve as a liaison between B. and his parents
**D.** Recall her own emotions when she was B.'s age

## Answer sheet

A B C D
1 ○○○○
2 ○○○○
3 ○○○○
4 ○○○○
5 ○○○○
6 ○○○○
7 ○○○○
8 ○○○○
9 ○○○○
10 ○○○○
11 ○○○○
12 ○○○○
13 ○○○○
14 ○○○○
15 ○○○○
16 ○○○○
17 ○○○○
18 ○○○○
19 ○○○○
20 ○○○○
21 ○○○○
22 ○○○○
23 ○○○○
24 ○○○○
25 ○○○○
26 ○○○○
27 ○○○○

## Answers and rationales

**1** Correct answer—**A**

Children who cannot cope with stress commonly act out their inse-curities in attention-getting ways. Behavior problems in children include attention deficit-hyperactivity disorder (characterized by inattentiveness and impulsive behavior), oppositional disorder (characterized by defiance of authority, angry acting-out behav-iors, and use of obscene language), and conduct disorder (charac-terized by persistent patterns of antisocial activity and disregard for behavioral norms). Signs of psychosis, such as autistic think-ing and loss of contact with reality, are not seen in persons with be-havioral disorders.

**2** Correct answer—**C**

A child with Tourette's syndrome—a tic disorder characterized by involuntary nonrhythmic motor movements and vocalizations—should not be given methylphenidate (Ritalin), a stimulant whose effect would worsen the symptoms. Therefore, the nurse should question the medication order immediately.

**3** Correct answer—**A**

Bulimia is an eating disorder characterized by a binge-purge cycle in which a person consumes large quantities of food, then purges (induces vomiting) to control her weight. The purging also re-lieves the abdominal distention associated with excessive eating and drinking. Conduct disorder is characterized by antisocial be-havior, not binging and purging activities. Although induced vom-iting is sometimes a characteristic of anorexia nervosa—an eating disorder marked by an intense aversion to weight gain and a fear of obesity, binging is not an aspect of this disorder. A gluttonous person consumes a large amount of food but typically does not in-duce vomiting.

**4** Correct answer—**B**

Unlike an anorexic patient, a bulimic patient typically has some in-sight into her behavior; she views binging and purging as abnor-mal but may be unable to control or stop the behavior. Despite this realization, the bulimic patient typically is unaware that her behav-ior is dangerous and can have serious physical consequences.

## 5 Correct answer—A

A bulimic patient tends to react impulsively, in contrast to an anorexic patient, who is more controlled. No specific personality traits, such as seriousness, have been associated with bulimia. However, personality differences are usually considered when treatment and interventions are planned. Intellectual abilities are not characteristically different from the norm in either group.

## 6 Correct answer—C

Telling the patient that she is not really hearing voices is a confrontational statement that will undoubtedly interfere with the development of a therapeutic nurse-patient relationship. Hallucinations are a defensive coping response to severe anxiety and are real to the patient who experiences them. Asking L. about possible drug use, what the voices say to her, and whether she has experienced hallucinations previously is appropriate and will provide the data needed to define problems, set goals, and plan interventions.

## 7 Correct answer—C

By informing L. that she sees no one in the room besides them, the nurse shares her own perception to assist L. with reality testing—the process of distinguishing subjective (internal) stimuli from objective (external) stimuli and making objective evaluations of one's environment. Responding with unnecessary abruptness ("You know that Daddy isn't in that chair") denies L.'s experience and is a less helpful reply. Reinforcing L.'s autistic perception ("I'll sit in another chair" or "Would Daddy like to go to the recreation hall?") is nontherapeutic because it does not encourage reality testing.

## 8 Correct answer—C

Inviting a calm, sensitive patient to join in on her conversation with L. enables the nurse to provide a supportive yet controlled environment as she introduces the patient to a new, potentially stressful behavior—relating to others. At this point, including a very outgoing person in the conversation probably would overwhelm L. and may increase her need for withdrawal. Because a withdrawn patient is unable to choose to interact with others, introducing her to a large group or letting her decide whether to interact with others probably will be unsuccessful.

**9** Correct answer—**A**

Infantile autism, which is commonly diagnosed before age 2½, is characterized by delayed developmental milestones, stereotyped behaviors (such as head banging and rocking), frequent crying, limited or no attempts at verbalization, and preference for solitary activities. Autism is differentiated from moderate retardation (marked by an IQ of 35 to 49) by the child's lack of social interaction and any form of communication. Antisocial personality, which is characterized by manipulation and disregard for social norms, generally is not diagnosed until late childhood or adolescence because some manipulation and challenging of norms is expected as a child strives for independence. Paranoid personality, typified by suspicion of the actions and motives of others, is a maladaptive coping pattern identifiable in late adolescence or early adulthood.

**10** Correct answer—**C**

Children such as T. require a safe, orderly, neutral environment to decrease the number of anxiety-provoking stimuli. Because an autistic child has an aversion to hugs and cuddling, the nurse must be cautious about the use of touch. Unless the mother-child relationship is extremely disturbed, the nurse should work with the family to care for the child. An autistic child usually is not hospitalized until late childhood (school-age or older), when the child's behavior may become unmanageable at home. Autism is treated through a holistic approach that may include medication (major tranquilizers), educational therapy (classroom experiences), and milieu therapy (manipulation of the environment to produce behavioral changes).

**11** Correct answer—**B**

Behavior modification—encouraging desired behaviors through positive reinforcement—is the best treatment approach for a young autistic child. Psychoanalysis and group therapy are appropriate for older children who have verbal skills. Behavior modification commonly is combined with play therapy in treating autistic children. Play therapy, which involves the use of toys and games to reveal a child's problems and fears, is especially effective with young children who are not yet able to verbally explore their feelings.

## 12 Correct answer—D

Encouraging T. to play with a ball is inappropriate because autistic children commonly are obsessively attached to objects, such as balls, and must be weaned from them. Treatment goals for an autistic child include maintaining contact with reality, developing self-concept, and accepting healthy nurturance. By encouraging the child to maintain contact with reality, the nurse can help him identify anxiety-producing stimuli and learn how to deal with them. As the child learns to handle daily challenges, his self-concept will improve. Even though an autistic child fears rejection and mistrusts nurturing role models, he has a great need for nurturing individuals. Helping the child accept nurturance allows this need to be met.

## 13 Correct answer—C

A child with disruptive behavior (conduct) disorder typically is witty, charming, and manipulative; he commits antisocial acts, such as arson and delinquency. Such a child is unable to recognize that his behavior is wrong and therefore does not benefit from punishment. Pervasive developmental disorder is an autistic condition; it may be classified as either infantile autism (diagnosed before age 2½) or childhood autism (diagnosed between ages 2½ and 12). Mental retardation is mental impairment indicated by an IQ of less than 70. Separation anxiety is excessive concern about separation from those to whom one is attached; it is most common in toddlers and preschoolers.

## 14 Correct answer—A

Storytelling and lying are characteristic of a child with a disruptive behavior disorder. The stories are typically an attempt to manipulate others and gain favor or privileges. Such storytelling is not an appeal for help or a way of belittling the nurse because the patient sees nothing wrong with his behavior. Delusions are indicative of psychosis, not antisocial behavior.

## 15 Correct answer—C

A patient with an antisocial (conduct) disorder manipulates others to get what he wants. If manipulation efforts are unsuccessful, the patient typically experiences increased anxiety that can lead to other manipulative actions, including suicide attempts. Managing such a patient requires providing a controlled environment and a consistent team approach. Such measures convey a sense of security and help to decrease anxiety. Breaking the rules is a sign of D.'s conduct disorder; the nurse must recognize this behavior as a manifestation of D.'s condition but should not accept it. D. would probably view threats to discharge him from the unit as a sign of his failed manipulation, which could lead to more manipulative behavior. A patient with a conduct disorder feels no guilt or remorse over misdeeds.

## 16 Correct answer—D

A patient with an antisocial (conduct) disorder typically is intelligent, with an above-average IQ, and uses his intelligence to manipulate others for personal gain. The primary deficit in such a patient is lack of emotional response; the patient views relationships primarily in light of whom he can control. He typically has a weak superego, resulting in a poor social conscience and lack of judgment.

## 17 Correct answer—C

To implement a behavior modification program effectively, all staff members must agree on the treatment plan. Consistency is essential to prevent the patient from manipulating the staff and to avoid sending mixed messages to the patient. Behavior modification focuses on treating current problem behaviors, not past events. Although a medical history may be useful, it is not essential in this case. Once staff members have agreed on the most appropriate treatment plan, they must set realistic goals and select a reward that is important to D to ensure its success.

## 18 Correct answer—C

Before discussing whether R. should be transferred to another school, the nurse should learn more about his behavior and the extent of his difficulties. The best way of gaining such information is to question the mother about R.'s behavior at home with his family. After obtaining a broader picture of the situation, the nurse can explore the mother's perceptions of how a change in schools would help her child. The nurse should avoid giving advice or voicing her opinion without a sufficient basis for such comments.

## 19 Correct answer—A

A thorough psychosocial assessment involves determining the patient's family dynamics, including how other family members view R.'s difficulties. Because R. is the focus of the assessment, the primary reason for conducting family interviews is to help the nurse better understand R.'s current behaviors. After the nurse has identified R.'s problems, treatment goals can be formulated and presented to the family for discussion. Family therapy is not indicated unless R.'s problems have caused so much stress that other family members are affected. If the initial diagnostic workup reveals such problems, a more thorough assessment can be conducted to identify family disruptions. Until a psychosocial assessment is completed and treatment plan developed, the nurse will find it difficult to explain how the family can help control R.'s behavior.

## 20 Correct answer—D

Anorexia nervosa is an eating disorder characterized by a body weight 15% below normal, an emaciated appearance, and amenorrhea, which typically occurs before weight loss is noticeable. Adolescent girls and young women age 12 to 28 are at highest risk for this condition. The mortality rate for anorexia is as high as 15%, and patients must be monitored closely for nutritional status, weight, and vital signs. Bulimia is an eating disorder evidenced by binging followed by self-induced vomiting; it is most common in women ages 17 to 23. Pica is a craving for substances that are not foods, such as dirt, clay, chalk, glue, starch, and hair. A compulsive eating disorder is one in which the patient consumes food even though she is not hungry.

## 21 Correct answer—D

A patient with anorexia nervosa typically is concerned about her appearance and maintains personal hygiene and grooming practices despite her illness; therefore, a nursing diagnostic category of *Dressing and grooming self-care deficit* is inapplicable. However, such a patient does have a severely distorted body image (*Body image disturbance*) and cannot effectively cope with how she views herself (*Ineffective individual coping*). She may describe herself as fat even when obviously emaciated and impose extreme self-control over food intake. She even may refuse to eat despite being hungry (*Altered nutrition, less than body requirements*).

## 22 Correct answer—**D**

Because an anorexic patient has an unrelenting fear of obesity coupled with a disturbed body image, using logic and reasoning to persuade K. to alter her behavior and eat would be ineffective. Behavior modification has proved to be an effective treatment for anorexic patients like K. This type of therapy depends on a consistent regimen to achieve positive results and to limit the patient's manipulative demands, which are used to try to avoid eating. Typically, the patient earns specific privileges for incremental weight gain and is allowed visitors once she has attained a predesignated weight. The nurse must take special precautions to control the patient's manipulative behavior, including constant and close observation at mealtimes to ensure that the patient eats all her food and does not hide it her napkin, give it to others, or discard it in a trash receptacle. The nurse also must observe the patient closely after meals to curtail self-induced vomiting. Psychotherapy can help the patient gain insight into her behavior and develop a positive body image and more adaptive coping skills.

## 23 Correct answer—**C**

A patient with anorexia nervosa is attempting to control at least one aspect her life—eating. Such a patient has underlying anxieties and strives to live up to her own expectations, not those of others or of weight and height charts. Peer pressure may prompt an adolescent to start a diet but does not contribute to anorexic behavior.

## 24 Correct answer—**B**

The nurse should suspect that B. is suffering from depression based on the fact that his behavior has persisted for 2 months and he has withdrawn from normal activities. The nurse should realize that although B. has experienced a serious loss, he has made some extreme changes in his life beyond the scope of normal grieving reactions. B.'s behavior is more than a fear of never loving again or a fear of failing; his symptoms are indicative of depression. Therefore, his problem is cause for concern and should not be viewed as inconsequential.

## 25 Correct answer—C

B.'s abuse of beer and marijuana can be viewed as indirect self-destructive behavior. If not halted, such behaviors can lead to death. Although many teenagers occasionally drink beer or experiment with marijuana, nightly drinking and smoking are signs of withdrawal behavior. Psychotic behavior is evidenced by loss of contact with reality and hallucinations or delusions; direct self-destructive behavior, such as suicide, presents an immediate threat to the patient's life. At this time, B. does not show any evidence of either psychotic or direct self-destructive behavior.

## 26 Correct answer—A

Drinking, drug abuse, and high-speed driving present a serious and immediate danger to B.'s life. His actions have moved beyond anxiety and simple depression to suicidal behavior, and he requires immediate interventions to protect himself and others and to halt his self-destructive path. These interventions may consist of a suicide contract (in which the patient agrees not to harm himself and promises to call or visit the center if he feels he cannot live up to the contract) or hospitalization. B. does not display any signs of psychosis.

## 27 Correct answer—C

The nurse should facilitate interaction between B. and his parents by fostering an environment in which they can feel free to express themselves. Siding with either B. or his parents may inhibit communication and prevent the nurse from working effectively with the family. For instance, if the nurse sides with B., his parents will feel attacked; if she sides with the parents, B. will feel isolated. Working with teenagers can evoke negative feelings related to the nurse's own adolescence, so the nurse must always remain alert for such responses. If such feelings arise, she should discuss them with someone, such as another psychiatric nurse, who can help her cope with any unresolved conflicts or issues (for example, an unresolved conflict between the nurse and her parents).

# CHAPTER 10

# Geriatric Disorders

# Questions

**1** In a nursing home, the primary purpose of a reminiscing group is to:

**A.** Reorient confused patients
**B.** Teach skills needed for independent living
**C.** Provide opportunities for physical activity
**D.** Meet patient needs for companionship and interaction

**2** When formulating a teaching plan for elderly patients, the nurse must recognize that older adults typically:

**A.** Resist new routines and behaviors
**B.** Have decreased memory and cognitive abilities
**C.** Require a slower-paced program of learning
**D.** Respond best to visual stimulation

## SITUATION

*A., age 75, is ready to be discharged from the hospital after treatment for a hip fracture suffered when she fell in her apartment. She is considering being transferred to a nursing home.*

*Questions 3 to 5 refer to this situation.*

**3** A. tells the nurse that her funds are limited and most nursing homes are expensive. She is debating how to solve this problem and asks what to do. Which response is most therapeutic?

**A.** "What possibilities have you thought about so far?"
**B.** "Why don't you move in with your sister so you can share expenses with her?"
**C.** "You should talk with your son and see what he says"
**D.** "I'd let the social worker worry about finding a place you can afford"

**4** A. asks her son about the possibility of living with him and his
family. Her son and daughter-in-law ask the nurse if they will be
able to meet A.'s needs in their home. The nurse can help them
make their decision by:

**A.** Having the physician explain the care that A. will need at home
**B.** Referring the couple to social services to evaluate their home
and review A.'s needs
**C.** Encouraging the couple to visit several nursing homes and
compare them with home care
**D.** Discussing A.'s current needs and what can be expected as she
recovers further

**5** After several lengthy discussions with the health care team and
her family, A. decides to move in with her son. On the day she is
to leave, she tells the nurse that she is still concerned about the arrangement. How should the nurse respond?

**A.** "Everything will be fine, so don't worry so much"
**B.** "If you are unsure about this, we can help you make other
arrangements"
**C.** "What part of the arrangements are you most concerned
about?"
**D.** "It's perfectly natural for you to be concerned. Think positively and it will work out"

## SITUATION

*K., a 69-year-old widow with no children, lives alone and visits
several local clinics and private physicians' offices for medical
care. A physician at one of the clinics refers her to the public
health nurse for evaluation of her home medication management
because she is not responding to medications as expected. During
a visit to the patient's home, the nurse discovers a large collection
of prescription and over-the-counter drugs in K.'s bathroom and
kitchen, some of which were prescribed for her husband several
years ago. After conducting a careful physical and mental assessment, the nurse determines that K. has a medication management
problem and that she appears depressed.*

*Questions 6 to 10 refer to this situation.*

**6** Which medications found in K.'s medicine cabinet do *not* contribute to depression?

**A.** Naproxen (Naprosyn) and diazepam (Valium)
**B.** Ibuprofen (Motrin) and clonidine patch (Catapres-TTS)
**C.** Acetylsalicylic acid (aspirin) and furosemide (Lasix)
**D.** Acetaminophen with codeine (Tylenol with Codeine) and cimetidine (Tagamet)

**7** K. tells the nurse that she has been feeling somewhat depressed recently. The nurse points out that medication mismanagement could be a contributing factor. Which approach should the nurse take when advising K. about her medications?

**A.** Tell K. to stop all but her blood pressure medication until she sees her physician again
**B.** Instruct K. to stop only the medications that can cause or contribute to depression
**C.** Ask the referring physician to take over K.'s primary care and provide new prescriptions
**D.** Call each physician listed on the prescription bottles and ask if K. should continue taking the medication

**8** K. and the nurse formulate a short-term goal stipulating that K. will return to the medical clinic for a more complete evaluation of her medications and possible depression. During her next home visit, K. tells the nurse that she tried to comply with the instructions for follow-up evaluation but encountered some frustrating obstacles and never got to see a physician.

K. relates to the nurse that a clerk at the medical clinic would not give her an appointment and advised her instead to "go to a nearby psychiatric clinic where they treated depressed people." At the psychiatric clinic, the receptionist told her that she needed a referral from her physician before she would be accepted as a patient. K. did not pursue the appointment further. At this time, the nurse should:

**A.** Call the referring physician to secure an appointment for K. at the medical clinic and a referral to the psychiatric clinic

**B.** Acknowledge K.'s problems and suggest ways to overcome them, then have K. call for an appointment while remaining with her

**C.** Tell K. that the appointment at the medical clinic is important and that she should call again and be firm when speaking with the clerk

**D.** Assume the role of patient advocate by calling the medical clinic and telling the clerk she was incorrect in referring K. to the psychiatric clinic, then obtaining an appointment for K. at the medical clinic

---

**9** K. is evaluated by a physician and a psychiatrist, and her medication orders are clarified. The psychiatrist diagnoses depression and orders desipramine (Norpramin). Desipramine is preferred over amitriptyline (Elavil) for patients such as K. because:

**A.** It is more potent and can be given in smaller doses
**B.** It is less expensive
**C.** It has fewer anticholinergic side effects
**D.** It interacts with fewer medications

---

**10** The public health nurse continues to follow up on K.'s progress. Which intervention is best for K.'s depression?

**A.** Offering frequent reassurance that things will get better
**B.** Relating the experiences of other persons in similar situations who have overcome depression
**C.** Ignoring the patient's depressed mood to discourage its continuation
**D.** Helping the patient to express her feelings of depression, grief, and anger

---

### SITUATION

*T., a 70-year-old widower who lives with his 80-year-old sister, remained active in community groups until the past 6 months. Recently, he began staying at home more often and started complaining about feeling fatigued and uninterested in outside activities. T.'s sister persuades him to go to the local health clinic for a checkup.*

*Questions 11 to 14 refer to this situation.*

**11** The nurse who assesses T. suspects that he is depressed based on which history statement?

**A.** "I take several naps a day, which usually helps me feel better"
**B.** "I don't know what it is, but I'm just not interested in anything any more. I feel too tired and down to be with people"
**C.** "Sometimes I worry about who will take care of my sister if something happens to me"
**D.** "One of my best friends died last month. That makes three this year who died"

**12** The nurse is concerned about T.'s depression and knows that the risk of suicide is high among older patients because:

**A.** They do not respond well to antidepressive medication
**B.** They usually do not respond to nonpharmacologic treatments for depression
**C.** They usually succeed on their first attempt at suicide
**D.** They typically take many different medications

**13** The physician prescribes imipramine (Tofranil) 25 mg t.i.d. for Mr. T. and schedules him for outpatient treatment at the mental health clinic. Before discharge, the nurse should advise T. to:

**A.** Refrain from eating yogurt and aged cheeses
**B.** Increase his fluid and sodium intake
**C.** Report symptoms of urine retention
**D.** Avoid over-the-counter cold medications

**14** After 3 weeks on imipramine, T. tells the mental health nurse that he is becoming forgetful and even lost his way home one day. Which nursing action is the priority at this time?

**A.** Reporting these symptoms to the physician for immediate evaluation
**B.** Telling T. to go out with friends until his confusion passes
**C.** Alerting T.'s sister that T. needs supervision at home
**D.** Explaining that the confusion is temporary and should decrease over time

## SITUATION

*L.O., age 70, was found by the police sitting in a local park during a heavy rainstorm. She was able to state her name but could not remember where she lived. She said she was waiting in the park for someone to take her home. The police took her to the emergency department of a nearby hospital. She was later identified by her husband, age 76, who reported her missing when she did not return home from the supermarket.*

*Questions 15 to 20 to this situation.*

**15** Mr. O. is worried about his wife. He says to the nurse, "Nothing like this has ever happened before. I hope she's not sick." Which response is most appropriate?

**A.** "Are you sure this is the first time she's had a problem like this? It's unusual that someone would just get lost like that"
**B.** "Don't worry. She's safe, and we will take care of her now"
**C.** "Has your wife shown other signs of confusion over the past year or so?"
**D.** "Before I can tell you whether she is sick, she'll need to undergo further examination and testing"

**16** L. is admitted to the medical unit for treatment of exposure. She tells the nurse, "I can't believe all this fuss. The park is a big place, you know. I was just trying to get my bearings straight when the police brought me here." L.'s comments reflect which defense mechanism?

**A.** Rationalization
**B.** Reaction formation
**C.** Sublimation
**D.** Intellectualization

**17** Further testing reveals that L. has Alzheimer's disease. Which symptom is *not* indicative of this disorder?

**A.** Aphasia
**B.** Apraxia
**C.** Agnosia
**D.** Akathisia

**18** L. is being discharged home. When teaching Mr. O. how to care for his wife at home, the nurse should give highest priority to L.'s:

**A.** Communication ability
**B.** Nutrition
**C.** Safety
**D.** Hygiene

**19** Mr. O. has heard that patients with Alzheimer's disease forget the names of people and objects in their environment. He asks the nurse what he can do to prevent this from happening to his wife. How should the nurse respond?

**A.** "Unfortunately, nothing will prevent this from happening. Your understanding and patience are most important"
**B.** "Putting labels on objects may help stimulate memory, especially for objects that are part of your wife's daily routine"
**C.** "Having your wife repeat the names of the objects she uses each day will help her to remember them"
**D.** "To avoid frustrating your wife, let her point to rather than name the items she wants"

**20** The nurse recognizes that caring for a family member with Alzheimer's disease can alter family processes. Which intervention is most appropriate in helping such families to cope?

**A.** Encouraging the family members to place the patient in a nursing home before the illness creates extreme hardship
**B.** Instructing the family members in the use medications to manage the patient's symptoms and behavior
**C.** Teaching the family members about the nature of Alzheimer's disease and how to cope with the patient's illness
**D.** Helping the family members through their mourning over the degeneration of their loved one

# Answer sheet

A B C D
1 ○○○○
2 ○○○○
3 ○○○○
4 ○○○○
5 ○○○○
6 ○○○○
7 ○○○○
8 ○○○○
9 ○○○○
10 ○○○○
11 ○○○○
12 ○○○○
13 ○○○○
14 ○○○○
15 ○○○○
16 ○○○○
17 ○○○○
18 ○○○○
19 ○○○○
20 ○○○○

## Answers and rationales

**1** Correct answer—**D**

Reminiscing groups allow older patients to recount their life experiences and share perceptions about a common theme. Participants in these groups are encouraged to discharge cognitive and emotional energy while meeting their needs for companionship and interaction. One way to encourage reminiscing is to ask group members to share experiences about a specific event, such as a holiday. The nurse should discourage participants from rambling or becoming preoccupied with disassociated (unconnected) thoughts during reminiscence sessions. Groups that focus on keeping patients oriented to time, place, and person using physical props (such as clocks) and on discussion of current events are known as reality orientation groups. These groups are useful for moderately to severely confused persons. Some groups in nursing home settings incorporate teaching the participants the skills needed for independent living; however, this is not the primary purpose of reminiscing groups. A reminiscing group does not provide opportunities for physical activity.

**2** Correct answer—**C**

Research has shown that older adults learn best when the teaching is slower-paced and they can learn at their own rate. Sensory changes, such as hearing loss and impaired vision, commonly result in the slowed thinking and response rate seen in many older patients. Older patients can and often do adapt to new routines and behaviors once they learn why the changes are needed. Therefore, repetition and a clear sense of how the information is useful to them is important to any teaching plan. Memory, cognitive abilities, adaptation skills, and personality traits remain relatively stable as people age and should have no bearing on the teaching plan. However, older patients often have visual deficits related to presbyopia and cataracts, and the teaching plan must take these factors into account.

**3** Correct answer—**A**

Helping A. to identify and examine possible alternatives is the most therapeutic response. The nurse should encourage the patient to remain active in decisions involving her care. Advising A. to move in with her sister or to talk with her son presumes that the nurse knows what is best for the patient and places the patient in a dependent position. Although the social worker also can help A.

explore possibilities, saying "I'd let the social worker worry about..." removes decision-making powers from the patient, which is where they belong.

**4** Correct answer—**D**

The nurse's role is to provide emotional support and factual information so the patient and her family can make an informed decision about A.'s future care. The nurse is in an excellent position to discuss the patient's immediate and long-term care needs. After explaining the situation to the family members, the nurse should refer them to other professionals, such as the patient's physician or a social service worker, who can provide additional information. Once the family understands the patient's needs, they can assess and evaluate their resources and make an appropriate decision. If the family decides that they cannot care for the patient themselves, the nurse should encourage them to visit local nursing homes.

**5** Correct answer—**C**

The nurse should encourage A. to express her feelings more fully. Asking the patient to identify which part of the arrangements she is concerned about will help A. to focus and explore her thoughts. Offering false reassurance ("Everything will be fine" or "Think positively") belittles the patient's feelings and offers no help. Offering assistance with other arrangements before clarifying the patient's concerns is premature and nontherapeutic.

**6** Correct answer—**C**

Many older patients take multiple medications that interact to produce or contribute to symptoms of depression. Acetylsalicylic acid (aspirin), an analgesic-antipyretic, and furosemide (Lasix), a diuretic used to treat edema related to congestive heart failure, do not contribute to depression. Naproxen (Naprosyn), a commonly prescribed anti-inflammatory drug, ibuprofen (Motrin), an antirheumatic agent, and acetaminophen with codeine (Tylenol with Codeine), an analgesic, can cause or contribute to depression in older patients. Diazepam (Valium), an antianxiety drug, should be used in reduced doses in older patients because they are more vulnerable to its side effects. Antianxiety agents, such as diazepam, are members of the same pharmacologic class as alcohol, which is a depressant. The clonidine patch (Catapres-TTS), an antihypertensive medication, can contribute to depression, insomnia, and anxiety. Cimetidine (Tagamet), a histamine antagonist used to treat and prevent duodenal ulcers, can cause confusion and depression in older adults.

## 7 Correct answer—C

The nurse should contact the physician who made the initial referral and request that he act as K.'s primary care source. The nurse then can review all of K.'s medications with the physician and ask him to write new prescriptions based on the patient's current needs. Instructing the patient to stop her medications until she sees her physician or to stop only those suspected of contributing to depression would be inappropriate. Medication management requires the intervention of a primary care physician to coordinate K.'s prescriptions; calling each of the prescribing physicians would not meet this objective.

## 8 Correct answer—B

The nurse should acknowledge the patient's frustration in trying to schedule the proper appointment at the clinic and teach her how to overcome such roadblocks should they occur again. By remaining with K. when she calls to make an appointment rather than calling for her, having the physician make the call, or having her call later when she is alone, the nurse provides the patient with another chance for success. The nurse should direct her interventions toward increasing the patient's self-care skills, independence, and feelings of control in this situation.

## 9 Correct answer—C

The tricyclic antidepressant desipramine (Norpramin) is preferred over amitriptyline (Elavil) for elderly patients because it has fewer anticholinergic side effects. It produces less sedation and orthostatic hypotension, which lowers the incidence of dizziness and decreases the potential for falls. Older patients generally require smaller doses of antidepressants and must be monitored carefully, especially for signs of cardiac arrhythmias. The dosage, cost, and drug interaction profile of despiramine do not differ markedly from those of other tricyclic antidepressants.

## 10 Correct answer—D

Nursing interventions for a depressed patient should be directed to facilitating the patient's expression of feelings. Such verbalization allows the patient to understand and cope with her feelings of depression, grief, and anger. The nurse can help by acknowledging and accepting the patient's feelings and encouraging their ventilation. Although the nurse should offer hope that the patient will feel better with treatment, she should avoid giving false reassurance. Doing so may cause the patient to believe that the nurse is not being honest about her condition and may lower the patient's trust in the nurse. A depressed patient typically is too self-centered and self-concerned to benefit from stories about other depressed persons. Ignoring the patient's depression does not provide an opportunity for the patient to discuss her feelings.

## 11 Correct answer—B

In an older adult, depression commonly is characterized by inactivity preceded by a lack of interest in previously enjoyable activities. T.'s statement clearly expresses his fatigue and general lack of interest. Although napping is common among older adults, those who are depressed tend to take frequent naps that do not leave them refreshed. Concerns about death and dying or who will take care of close relatives are not unusual and are not a sign of depression unless the patient begins to ruminate or demonstrates obsessive tendencies, such as constantly thinking or speaking about the subject.

## 12 Correct answer—C

Statistics have shown that adults over age 65 account for more than 25% of the reported suicides in the United States and that most of those in this age-group who attempt suicide succeed on their first attempt; older men are at a particularly high risk. Therefore, the nurse should consider any older adult with depression a suicide risk. Depressed elderly patients do respond to antidepressive medication and other treatment modalities. However, diagnosis of depression can be difficult because the condition may be masked by preexisting physical disabilities or because the clinician may be inexperienced in recognizing it. Medication management can be complicated by the multiple medications taken by many elderly patients, which increases the risk for drug interactions. Although taking multiple medications does not increase the risk of suicide, special attention is needed in selecting drugs and dosages to minimize depressive side effects.

## 13 Correct answer—C

Because imipramine (Tofranil) can cause urine retention, the nurse must instruct T. to report any signs of this side effect, including abdominal distention and delayed micturition. She should advise the patient to drink at least 6 glasses of fluid each day and to encourage urination by relaxation techniques or running warm water over his genitals. If these approaches are unsuccessful, the patient should notify the physician immediately. Unlike monoamine oxidase inhibitors and other tricyclic antidepressants, imipramine has no food or over-the-counter drug restrictions. If the patient were taking lithium, he would be encouraged to increase his fluid and sodium intake to maintain proper lithium blood levels.

## 14 Correct answer—A

The nurse should alert the physician immediately because T. may be experiencing an anticholinergic side effect of the tricyclic antidepressant therapy. Symptoms include confusion and disorientation that may resemble organic brain disease. The physician can make a differential diagnosis by administering 1 to 2 mg of physostigmine (Antilirium) I.M. Physostigimine will temporarily reverse the symptoms if they are caused by imipramine. After Mr. T. has been evaluated by the physician, the nurse should inform him and his sister of the need for caution and supervision until the medication's side effects have abated. Although confusion is a common side effect of antidepressant therapy, telling the patient or his sister that the confusion is temporary would be inappropriate; the patient could have another underlying organic disorder that manifests as confusion.

## 15 Correct answer—C

The nurse should try to gather additional data about when L.'s confusion and disorientation first began. The onset of major degenerative disorders, such as Alzheimer's disease, usually is insidious, with symptoms occurring but often denied by the patient and family members for 1 to 2 years before more advanced disease is apparent. Information about earlier signs of confusion can help determine the diagnosis. The nurse should be sensitive to Mr. O.'s feelings and concern and should not abruptly challenge his perception or offer empty reassurance that he need not worry. Although the patient probably will require a thorough examination and further testing to determine the cause of her disorientation, the nurse should concentrate on gathering data to help the physician diagnose the problem and should avoid alarming the patient's husband.

## 16 Correct answer—**A**

L. is using rationalization to explain her confusion and disorientation. Older patients often attempt to cover up and make excuses for lapses and incidents of confusion to preserve self-esteem and deny symptoms. Reaction formation is the manifestation of behavior that is the opposite of the patient's true feelings, such as expressing a desire to enter a nursing home when this is not the case. Sublimation is a healthy defense mechanism whereby the patient satisfies unacceptable impulses by channeling them into acceptable behaviors—for example, becoming involved in volunteer work instead of acting on sexual impulses. Intellectualization is a defense mechanism in which the patient separates his feelings and thoughts about a situation and talks about the event without emotion—for example, stating the reasons why moving to a new home is a good idea while denying the feelings of loss associated with such a move.

## 17 Correct answer—**D**

Akathisia, or motor restlessness, is not a symptom of Alzheimer's disease. It is a side effect of many neuroleptic drugs and is evidenced by anxiety and restlessness that range from inner disquiet to an inability to sit still. Signs of Alzheimer's disease include aphasia (loss of language ability), apraxia (inability to perform previously known purposeful activities, such as dressing and toileting), and agnosia (difficulty in recognizing everyday objects and persons and, eventually, close relatives and loved ones). The onset of Alzheimer's disease is gradual and includes such symptoms as progressive memory loss, impaired judgment, decreased attention span, and inappropriate social behavior.

## 18 Correct answer—**C**

Safety should be the highest priority when caring for a patient such as L., who has already wandered off once and may do so again. Her impaired judgment and confusion increase the potential for injury and must be addressed by her family. The nurse should teach the family members how to ensure L.'s safety, such as by supervising her activity, decreasing hazards in the home (for example, locking up medications, tools, and cleaning agents), assessing neighborhood hazards, having her wear an identification bracelet, and installing alarms on exit doors in the home. The family must be prepared to deal with L.'s communication limitations by such means as keeping choices simple and using brief, direct statements or orienting statements. The family also must learn how to meet L.'s hygiene needs (such as bathing her and taking her to the bathroom regularly) and nutrition needs (such as serving nutritional snacks and maintaining her fluid intake).

## 19 Correct answer—B

During the onset of Alzheimer's disease, the patient may be able to recall familiar objects more easily if they are labeled. Structuring the environment in this way may stimulate long-term memory, at least for a time. Although the process of memory loss, aphasia, and agnosia cannot be reversed, the patient and her family members can continue to use memory-improving techniques, such as labeling objects, to reduce frustration. Having the patient name each object she uses may upset her as she finds it harder and harder to attach meaning to names. Family members should encourage the patient to maintain the skills and activities she can still perform rather than promote dependency prematurely.

## 20 Correct answer—C

An important role of the nurse in working with family members of patients with Alzheimer's disease is to educate them about the illness. Family members need to understand the nature of the disease, how it may progress, and what they can expect. The nurse should teach them how to manage the patient as well as how to cope with their own stress. When families must decide whether to place the patient in a nursing home, the nurse's role is to help the family understand all aspects of the decision, not to encourage nursing home placement. To date, drug therapy has been unsuccessful in managing Alzheimer's symptoms. However, ongoing research is investigating the use of the vasodilator cyclandelate (Cyclospasmol) and drugs to correct neurotransmitter deficiencies. Later, as the patient becomes more incapacitated and dysfunctional, the nurse can help support the family during their mourning.

# CHAPTER 11

# Comprehensive
# Examination

## Questions

**1** A primary difference between nursing models of psychiatric care and the psychosocial, behavioral, and medical models of psychiatric care is that the nursing models:

**A.** Focus on the person as an individual
**B.** Incorporate a holistic view of the person
**C.** Center on health instead of illness
**D.** Have a psychosocial not psychobiologic perspective

**2** Which nursing theorist developed a model for the therapeutic nurse-patient relationship that provided the first systematic theoretical framework for psychiatric nursing?

**A.** Peplau
**B.** Leininger
**C.** Orem
**D.** Rogers

**3** When assessing and recording a patient's mental status, a nurse must differentiate between observations and inferences. Which statement is based on observation?

**A.** "The patient prefers to remain dirty and disheveled and does not bother to shower in the morning"
**B.** "The patient likes to antagonize patients and staff members by refusing to shower"
**C.** "The patient does not respond to requests by staff members to shower and attend to personal grooming"
**D.** "The patient demonstrates negative behavior (refusal to shower) related to his need to control the environment"

**4** A therapeutic nurse-patient relationship is one in which:

**A.** The nurse sets the priorities and goals using the nursing process
**B.** The nurse permits the patient to establish the direction of the interactions
**C.** The nurse and the patient meet each other's needs
**D.** The nurse plans interactions to help the patient meet his needs

**5** Most therapeutic interaction with a patient occurs during which phase of the nurse-patient relationship?

**A.** Preinteraction
**B.** Introduction or orientation
**C.** Working
**D.** Termination

**6** A newly admitted patient tells the nurse that he had a fight with his wife 2 days ago and that yesterday, on his way home from work, he decided it would be thoughtful to buy her the emerald ring she always wanted. Which ego defense mechanism is this patient using?

**A.** Displacement
**B.** Rationalization
**C.** Projection
**D.** Undoing

**7** Three-year-old J. is admitted to the pediatric unit. The nurse notes that J. will drink fluids only through a bottle even though his mother states that he has been drinking from a cup for the past 9 months. The nurse concludes that the child is using the ego defense mechanism of:

**A.** Denial
**B.** Regression
**C.** Repression
**D.** Sublimation

**8** A., who is pursuing a nursing degree only to please her parents, is nominated for senior nursing class president. In her campaign speech, she speaks sincerely about how professional nursing is the best possible career choice. A.'s behavior is an example of which ego defense mechanism?

**A.** Reaction formation
**B.** Identification
**C.** Compensation
**D.** Denial

**9** A patient with a large duodenal ulcer is told that she must follow a bland diet. When her teenage children bring home a pepperoni pizza, she states, "How wonderful. My physician said that I have a small ulcer but that I can eat anything I want." The patient is probably using which ego defense mechanism?

A. Splitting
B. Compensation
C. Rationalization
D. Denial

**10** A young male patient recovering from a cholecystectomy is undergoing psychotherapy to help him cope with his ego-dystonic homosexuality. One morning, he emphatically whispers to the nurse, "You must get my room changed. My roommate is making homosexual gestures toward me." The patient is using the ego defense mechanism of:

A. Displacement
B. Intellectualization
C. Projection
D. Identification

**11** Which test is most widely used to aid in diagnosing depression?

A. Coagulation profile and protein uptake test
B. Dexamethasone suppression test
C. Theophylline level test
D. Follicle-stimulating hormone and thyroid-stimulating hormone levels test

**12** Which type of hallucination is an initial symptom of alcoholic hallucinosis?

A. Tactile
B. Olfactory
C. Auditory
D. Visual

**13** Which statement most accurately describes Alcoholics Anonymous (AA)?

**A.** AA is a complex organization in which professional counselors help alcoholic persons with their problems
**B.** AA consists of local, loosely organized groups in which alcoholic persons help each other to stay sober
**C.** AA is an organization that focuses on teaching the public about alcoholism
**D.** AA works indirectly with alcoholic persons through research and education programs

**14** Which commonly administered psychiatric medication has an absolute maximum dosage?

**A.** Chlorpromazine (Thorazine)
**B.** Alprazolam (Xanax)
**C.** Lithium (Lithane)
**D.** Thioridazine (Mellaril)

**15** Any nurse who administers antipsychotic medications must be alert for early signs and symptoms of:

**A.** Neuroleptic malignant syndrome
**B.** Pseudoparkinsonism
**C.** Sedation
**D.** Blurred vision

**16** The physician may prescibe amino acid therapy for a cocaine abuser to:

**A.** Compensate for poor nutritional habits
**B.** Restore depleted neurotransmitters
**C.** Help detoxify residual cocaine
**D.** Reduce agitation

**17** Which foods are contraindicated for a patient taking tranylcypromine (Parnate)?

**A.** Whole grain cereals and bagels
**B.** Chicken livers, Chianti wine, and beer
**C.** Oranges and vodka
**D.** Chicken, rice, and apples

---

### SITUATION

*B., an extremely withdrawn 19-year-old engineering student, is admitted to the psychiatric unit. The physician has prescribed chlorpromazine 150 mg q.i.d., and B. has already received two doses.*

*Questions 18 to 27 refer to this situation.*

---

**18** B. paces the halls and makes many trips to the water fountain. If this behavior continues, which nursing diagnosis is most applicable?

A. Urge incontinence related to excessive fluid intake
B. Impaired adjustment related to anxiety
C. Fluid volume excess related to attempts to relieve dry mouth
D. Fatigue related to continual pacing

---

**19** Which nursing intervention is most appropriate for B.'s repeated trips to the water fountain?

A. Tell B. that he may drink water only once each hour
B. Offer B. sugarless gum to chew instead of drinking water
C. Take B. to his room and suggest that he watch television
D. Provide B. with emotional support while unobtrusively supervising his behavior

---

**20** B. reports that he hears the voice of his brother, who was recently killed in an auto accident, telling him to hang himself so the two brothers can be together. How should the nurse respond?

A. "That's impossible. Dead people can't talk"
B. "We'll be placing you on suicide precautions so you won't act on his command"
C. "Tell me what your brother was like"
D. "Killing yourself doesn't guarantee that you'll join your brother"

**21** B. has been receiving chlorpromazine 150 mg q.i.d. for 2 days. After lunch, he rises from his chair and begins to sway, then reaches out to take hold of the table and sits down. When asked to describe what happened, he mumbles that he does not know. The priority nursing action is to:

**A.** Continue to observe B. from a distance
**B.** Reorient B. to person, place, and time
**C.** Encourage B. to return to his room
**D.** Assess B.'s blood pressure while he is sitting and standing

**22** Which nursing action would best help B. while he is dizzy?

**A.** Teaching him to rise slowly
**B.** Providing him with one-to-one supervision
**C.** Having him remain in bed
**D.** Calling his physician

**23** After 7 days on chlorpromazine, B. shows signs of occasional drooling, stiff movements, and hand tremors. These signs probably indicate:

**A.** An appropriate medication dosage
**B.** An excessive medication dosage
**C.** Extrapyramidal side effects
**D.** Severe drug toxicity

**24** The most appropriate nursing action for B.'s drooling and stiff movements is to:

**A.** Notify the physician
**B.** Teach B. relaxation techniques
**C.** Withhold the next dose of medication
**D.** Reassure B. that the symptoms will disappear when his body adjusts to the medication

**25** After 3 weeks in the hospital, B. improves sufficiently to go home for the weekend. The nurse gives him a 2-day supply of medication, then instructs him to:

**A.** Avoid contact with anyone who has an upper respiratory tract infection
**B.** Spend at least 1 hour each day outside
**C.** Avoid such foods as aged cheese and pickled herring
**D.** Avoid driving a car and operating machinery

**26** As B. improves, he is allowed to leave the hospital for several days at a time. One day, he goes skiing and returns with a severe sun burn. Which nursing intervention is most appropriate?

**A.** Ask B. to discuss his proposed activities with staff members before he leaves the hospital
**B.** Advise B. to use a sunscreen before going out in the sun
**C.** Provide B. with a ski mask for the next time he goes skiing
**D.** Have B. take large doses of vitamin D before exposure to the sun

**27** One of the patient goals established for B. is that he will understand the potential interactions between his prescribed medication and other substances. The nurse determines that B. has achieved this goal when he states:

**A.** "I should use enemas instead of cathartics"
**B.** "I should not drink alcoholic beverages"
**C.** "I can drink as much coffee and tea as I like"
**D.** "I will get a skin rash if I take antibiotics"

---

### SITUATION

*S., age 34, arrives at the hospital anxious, crying, and shaking. She tells the nurse that she began feeling depressed and apathetic 18 months ago, when her husband told her he wanted a divorce. A biochemist, she has worked long hours and extra shifts to put her husband through law school. After her husband left and began divorce proceedings, she became withdrawn and intensely unhappy with feelings of constant tiredness, grief, hopelessness, and worthlessness. The physician diagnoses major depression.*

*Questions 28 to 31 refer to this situation.*

**28** The nurse knows that sadness typically accompanies grief and depression. Which other affect changes indicate major depression?

**A.** Fear, timidity, and lack of interest in surroundings
**B.** Withdrawal, negative attitude, and little or no eye contact
**C.** Lack of incentive, dominating personality, and defensiveness
**D.** Irritability, apathy, and self-doubt

**29** The physician prescribes phenelzine sulfate (Nardil) 15 mg P.O., followed by 15 mg P.O. t.i.d. to be continued at home. The nurse should instruct S. to do all of the following *except:*

**A.** Avoid eating aged cheeses, liver, and yogurt
**B.** Take the medication 1 hour before meals
**C.** Limit alcoholic beverages to white wine only
**D.** Avoid driving a car

**30** The nurse recognizes that S. needs help coping with her feelings of loss and grief related to the end of her marriage. The nurse can assist the patient best by:

**A.** Telling her to forget the past and make a new start for herself
**B.** Encouraging her to engage in group therapy with others who have similar problems
**C.** Encouraging her to discuss her loss and offering comfort and support
**D.** Reminding her that time heals all wounds

**31** S. is afraid to face her feelings or show any emotions about the breakup of her marriage. She says that reliving old memories and the pain she suffered makes her feel worse. The nurse can help the patient handle this part of the grieving process by:

**A.** Telling S. that she will not cry forever, permanently lose control, or go crazy if she grieves
**B.** Reflecting back what S. has said so she can hear what she is expressing
**C.** Asking S. if she needs additional medication during this difficult time
**D.** Reassuring S. that her feelings of guilt about her failed marriage will end soon

## SITUATION

*L. arrives at the well-baby clinic with her 6-month-old son for a routine checkup. In reviewing the infant's chart, the nurse discovers that during a previous visit, L. stated jokingly that her son does not like her.*

*Questions 32 to 35 refer to this situation.*

**32** Which assessment finding is considered abnormal for a 6-month-old infant?

A. Responds to name
B. Appears indifferent to nurse's actions
C. Reaches for stethoscope
D. Fidgets in mother's arms

**33** The nurse asks L. to describe her son's usual behavior. Which statement should lead the nurse to suspect autism?

A. "He talks or babbles constantly"
B. "He cries frequently to be picked up"
C. "He lies quietly in his crib for hours"
D. "He watches everything that goes on around him"

**34** The nurse asks L. to describe what her son does that makes her think he does not like her. Which response indicates deviant social development?

A. "When I hold him, he just lies there or stiffens up. He doesn't cuddle or smile at me much"
B. "He cries a lot, and sometimes it's hard to quiet him down"
C. "He seems to like my mother more than me. He gets excited, smiles, and babbles for her but not for me"
D. "He wants to be held all day"

**35** The nurse refers L. to the child guidance clinic for further assessment and evaluation of her son's behavior. The nurse should explain to L. that:

A. Her son should be cured by early intervention
B. Her son's maladaptive behavior should decrease with early treatment
C. Her son needs to be cuddled properly
D. Her son can be taught to be spontaneous and responsive

## SITUATION

*B., a 60-year-old widow, is admitted to the psychiatric unit with a diagnosis of unipolar affective disorder.*

*Questions 36 to 41 refer to this situation.*

**36** Which psychotropic medication will the physician most likely prescribe for B.?

A. Lorazepam (Ativan)
B. Imipramine (Tofranil)
C. Thiothixene (Navane)
D. Alprazolam (Xanax)

**37** The nurse should advise B. that she can expect a full therapeutic response to her medication within:

A. 1 week
B. 7 to 10 days
C. 2 weeks
D. 3 to 4 weeks

**38** B.'s depression does not improve with antidepressant medication, and the physician orders electroconvulsive therapy (ECT). ECT's mechanism of action is:

A. Related to the patient's perception of ECT as a well-deserved punishment
B. Unclear at present
C. Related to an increased production of chemicals in the brain
D. Similar to that of antidepressant drugs

**39** When preparing B. for ECT, the nurse should ensure that all of the following have been done *except:*

A. The patient has signed an informed consent document
B. The patient and her family have been instructed about the ECT procedure
C. The patient has undergone a thorough medical evaluation
D. The patient has received lithium

**40** Nursing preparations for a patient undergoing ECT are similar to those used in:

A. Physical therapy
B. Neurologic examinations
C. General anesthesia
D. Cardiac stress testing

**41** During or after the ECT procedure, B. may experience all of the following side effects *except:*

A. Disrupted short- and long-term memory
B. Transient confusional state
C. Headache
D. Backache

---

### SITUATION

*C., a 28-year-old with schizophrenia, is admitted to the acute psychiatric unit. He was brought to the hospital by the police, who found him lying naked on a bench in an urban park. The officers report that C.'s lips were moving constantly as if he were in conversation.*

*Questions 42 to 47 refer to this situation.*

**42** When communicating with C., the nurse should initially:

A. Remain silent and wait for C. to speak first
B. Talk with C. as she would talk with a healthy person
C. Allow C. to do all the talking
D. Speak to C. using simple, concrete language

**43** C. mentions that voices are telling him that he is in danger and that he will be safe only if he stays in his room and avoids "zoids." How should the nurse respond?

A. "I understand that these voices are real to you, but I want you to know that I don't hear them"
B. "Don't worry. I won't let anything happen to you here"
C. "What else can you tell me about the voices?"
D. "Many patients hear voices when they come here. The voices will go away when you get better"

**44** During the admission interview, C. indicates that he has been taking medication to help eliminate the voices. Further assessment reveals that he is photosensitive and has a parkinsonian tremor. These effects are commonly experienced by patients on which drug therapy?

A. Diazepam (Valium)
B. Trifluoperazine (Stelazine)
C. Oxazepam (Serax)
D. Meprobomate (Miltown)

**45** Which nursing intervention is inappropriate for a hallucinating patient?

A. Determining which needs the hallucinations meet and attempting to meet those needs in other ways
B. Responding positively to discussions of specific hallucinations
C. Orienting the patient to reality
D. Responding positively to the patient's periods of reality

**46** C. tells the nurse that another male patient has been flirting with him and wants to begin a sexual relationship. The nurse knows that all of the following statements are true *except:*

A. C. may have a gender identity problem
B. C. probably is using projection to cope with his anxiety
C. C. is experiencing delusions of grandeur
D. C. may fear his own sexuality

**47** Which nursing intervention can best help to decrease C.'s anxiety about his sexuality?

A. Increase the dosage of his antipsychotic medication
B. Restrict him to his room except for meals
C. Confront him with the reality of his feelings
D. Assign him to a private room

## SITUATION

*J., a 36-year-old accountant, is brought to the psychiatric unit by his wife, who reports that he recently began cutting off his interpersonal relationships and expressing fears that his boss wants him fired. He has accused his wife of having an affair with his boss and refuses to eat any of the meals she prepares. The only way J.'s wife could get him to the hospital today was to persuade him to allow an objective physician to judge their situation.*

*Questions 48 to 51 refer to this situation.*

**48** When the nurse suggests hospitalization, J. states, "I should have known that they would have gotten to you first." Which response by the nurse is most therapeutic?

A. "What makes you think someone has gotten to me?"
B. "I'm your nurse, and I'm here to help you"
C. 'You seem very suspicious of me. Are you?"
D. "I've never met your wife or your boss before"

**49** After 1 week on the unit, J. tells the nurse that he will not attend his group therapy session because a student nurse is there to spy on him. Which response by the nurse is best?

A. "If you come to your therapy session, I'll take you for a walk outside afterward"
B. "What makes you think she's spying on you?"
C. "It is my understanding that student nurses attend therapy sessions as part of their education"
D. "Come to therapy. I'll protect you"

**50** The nurse observes J. pushing his food around on his plate but not actually eating anything. She also notices him carefully watching the other patients at his table eat their lunch. What action should the nurse take to help J. meet his nutritional needs?

A. Sit with J. and encourage him to eat his lunch
B. Ask J. if something is wrong with his meal
C. Continue to allow J. to observe his tablemates
D. Provide J. with packaged, high-protein, between-meal snacks

**51** J. is given a complicated paint-by-numbers project for his occupational therapy. The nurse knows that suspicious patients should be given activities involving a high level of concentration because:

A. They need to be challenged by various tasks
B. They lose interest easily if not concentrating
C. They will have less time for delusional thinking
D. They will have less need for physically acting out

## SITUATION

*D., age 8, is referred to the child guidance clinic by the school nurse because he cannot sit still, continually disrupts the class, rarely finishes assignments, and frequently fights with classmates.*

*Questions 52 to 55 refer to this situation.*

**52** Psychological testing reveals that D. has an attention deficit disorder (ADD) with hyperactivity. The nurse knows that this disorder is characterized by:

A. Impulsiveness and inattentiveness
B. Adaptive behavior deficits and a below-average intelligence
C. A lack of regard for authority and the rights of others
D. Impaired thinking and emotional instability

**53** Which nursing diagnosis is most applicable for D. at this time?

A. Ineffective family coping related to ineffective parenting
B. Potential for injury related to impulsivity
C. Impaired verbal communication related to mutism
D. Altered thought processes related to impaired reality

**54** The physician determines that D. will benefit most from drug therapy. Which drug classification is most commonly prescribed for children with ADD?

A. Sedatives
B. Antidepressants
C. Cerebral stimulants
D. Antianxiety agents

**55** Which medication side effect is typically the greatest concern of parents with children with ADD?

A. Dizziness
B. Headache
C. Increased appetite
D. Delayed physical growth

## SITUATION

*J., a 14-year-old boy with a history of truancy, shoplifting, fighting, and running away from home, is remanded by family court to a residential treatment center.*

*Questions 56 to 59 refer to this situation.*

**56** Which approach by the nurse would be best when interacting with J.?

A. Passive friendliness
B. Active friendliness
C. Kind firmness
D. Laissez-faire

**57** J.'s 16-year-old sister resists attending family therapy. She states, "This is just what I need on top of all the other embarrassments. Now my friends will think I'm crazy, too." How should the nurse respond?

A. "Your brother should be more important to you than your friends"
B. "Are you afraid we'll find something wrong with you also?"
C. "Don't be silly. How will your friends know?"
D. "It sounds as if things haven't been easy for you"

**58** J.'s conduct disorder is of the unsocialized aggressive type. Management of such a patient primarily is directed to:

A. Preventing peer-influenced behaviors
B. Decreasing his hostility toward others
C. Fostering a sense of accountability for his behavior
D. Decreasing self-mutilating behavior

**59** If J. does not respond to therapy now, as an adult he probably will be diagnosed as having:

A. Borderline personality disorder
B. Schizoid personality disorder
C. Antisocial personality disorder
D. Passive-aggressive personality disorder

## SITUATION

*M., age 25, is found sitting on the floor of the bathroom in the day treatment clinic with moderate lacerations to both wrists. Sur-*

*rounded by broken glass, she sits staring blankly at her bleeding wrists while staff members call for an ambulance.*

*Questions 60 to 64 refer to this situation.*

**60** How should the nurse approach M. initially?

**A.** Enter the room quietly and move beside M. to assess her injuries

**B.** Call for staff backup before entering the room and restraining M.

**C.** Move as much glass away from M. as possible and quietly sit next to her

**D.** Approach M. slowly while speaking in a calm voice, calling her name and telling her that the nurse is here to help her

**61** M. is taken to the hospital and admitted on an emergency basis for 72 hours, as provided by state law. M. says to the admitting nurse, "I'm not staying here. I was a little upset and did a stupid thing. I want to leave." Which response is most appropriate?

**A.** "Unfortunately, you have no right to leave at this time. You must be evaluated further"

**B.** "Cutting your wrists certainly was a stupid thing to do. What were you trying to accomplish anyway?"

**C.** "You have been admitted on an emergency basis and can be held up to 72 hours. You have the right to consult a lawyer about your admission"

**D.** "I can see you're upset. Why don't you try to relax. You can explain to the physician what upset you. If what you say is true, you'll be released sooner"

**62** Determining M.'s suicide potential during the mental status examination involves assessing several factors, the most significant of which is her:

**A.** History of previous suicide attempts

**B.** Suicide plan

**C.** Emotional state

**D.** Self-esteem

**63** M. is placed on suicide precautions, which include constant observation. When the nurse accompanies her to the bathroom, M. complains, "I can't believe this. I can't even go to the bathroom without being watched. How would you like to have me watching you go to the toilet?" Which response by the nurse is best?

**A.** "I'm sure I wouldn't like it very much, but then I didn't try to hurt myself"
**B.** "I'm sorry but these are the rules. Someone must be with you at all times"
**C.** "If it's more comfortable for you, I can stand right outside as long as the door is open. Would you agree to that?"
**D.** "I would probably feel uncomfortable too, but ensuring your safety is my first priority. I must stay in the room with you"

**64** After 5 days of hospitalization, M. is to be discharged and treated on an outpatient basis at the day treatment clinic. During the discharge planning, the nurse should set as a priority short-term goal that M. will:

**A.** Identify support systems to help manage stress
**B.** Verbalize feelings of shame regarding her suicide attempt
**C.** Demonstrate an uplifted mood and optimism about the future
**D.** Admit that her wrist slashing was an attention-seeking behavior and not a true suicide attempt

---

### SITUATION

*A.G., a 32-year-old architect, arrives at the local mental health center with his wife, who explains to the admitting nurse that over the past month her husband has been exhibiting elevated mood, insomnia, and increasing hyperactivity and has lost 20 lb (9.1 kg). Mrs. G. tells the nurse that she finally decided her husband needed help when he drew up plans to renovate their home, spent $60,000 on supplies, and announced that he was doing all the work himself. His admitting diagnosis is bipolar disorder of the manic type.*

*Questions 65 to 71 refer to this situation.*

**65** A. is taken to a private room on the psychiatric unit, where the nurse is to complete the admission interview. She finds A. pacing restlessly in his room and speaking rapidly about how he is going to have the biggest and best house in town. How should the nurse approach A. while he is in a hyperactive state?

**A.** Tell him that he must sit down quietly while she completes the admission interview
**B.** Walk around with him as he paces, asking questions whenever he quiets down
**C.** Sit down with him and have him attempt to focus on answering a few essential questions
**D.** Postpone the admission interview until he can concentrate better

**66** The physician prescribes lithium (Lithane) 600 mg P.O. stat followed by 300 mg q.i.d. The nurse should:

**A.** Question the prescription
**B.** Ask the physician to prescribe chlorpromazine (Thorazine) as needed for agitation
**C.** Suggest that an antiparkinsonian drug be administered concurrently
**D.** Administer the lithium as ordered

**67** The history reveals that A. has been overweight for the past several years. Having lost 20 lb in the previous month, he now is 15 lb (6.8 kg) above the recommended weight for his height. Which intervention is best at this time?

**A.** Monitor A.'s intake, output, and weight on a daily basis
**B.** Offer A. finger foods and high-protein drinks
**C.** Have A. eat a regular diet but do not offer supplements
**D.** Encourage A. to exercise to lose the additional 15 lb

**68** The day after admission, the nurse finds A. in the dayroom sketching plans for renovating the psychiatric unit. He has an audience of 10 other patients and has them moving furniture back and forth across the room. The nurse should:

**A.** Do nothing and continue to observe A. and the other patients for signs of increased agitation
**B.** Confront A. and remind him that he is a patient, not a decorator
**C.** Encourage the other patients to criticize A.'s grandiose plans
**D.** Request that A. pick up his plans, then accompany him to his room

**69** A. sleeps only 1 to 2 hours at night and not at all during the day. Which action would *not* promote rest in a patient who is having trouble sleeping?

**A.** Administering a sedative at night as ordered
**B.** Encouraging a short nap during the day
**C.** Teaching the patient relaxation techniques
**D.** Allowing the patient to talk quietly with a staff member when he has trouble sleeping

**70** After 1 week on the unit, the nurse hears A. arguing with P., another patient on the unit who borrowed one of his shirts without permission. A. begins shouting, "I have thousands of shirts. I am the Shirt King. Ask and you shall receive. Thou shalt not steal. What's mine is yours." How should the nurse respond?

**A.** "A., it sounds as if you're angry with P. for borrowing your shirt without asking. What should he do the next time he wants to borrow something from you?"
**B.** "I can understand how upsetting it is to have P. take your shirt. P., you know it is against the rules to take other people's things without asking"
**C.** "A., you are losing control of yourself and making no sense. What are you trying to say to P.?"
**D.** "A., go back to your room and calm down. You can talk this over with P. later when you're less upset"

**71** After 3 weeks on lithium therapy within the unit's structured environment, A. is given a weekend pass to go home. He calls the unit at 2:15 p.m. on Saturday to tell the nurse that he forgot to take his 1:00 p.m. dose. The nurse should tell him to:

**A.** Omit the 1:00 dose and take his next regular dose at 5:00 p.m.
**B.** Omit the 1:00 dose and double his 5:00 p.m. dose
**C.** Take the 1:00 dose now and the next dose, as scheduled, at 5:00 p.m.
**D.** Take the 1:00 dose now and the next dose 2 hours later than planned

---

### SITUATION

*L., age 17, is brought to the emergency department by four of his friends. He is extremely agitated and combative, hallucinating and shouting obscenities at everyone in the room. His friends report that they were at a party where L. must have taken some "bad stuff," which they could not identify. The tentative diagnosis is acute toxic psychosis.*

*Questions 72 to 74 refer to this situation.*

---

**72** The management of L. in the emergency department should be primarily directed toward:

**A.** Controlling withdrawal symptoms
**B.** Sedating the patient
**C.** Waiting for the drug's effects to wear off
**D.** Maintaining the safety of the patient and others

---

**73** Which physical assessment finding indicates that L. ingested phencyclidine (PCP) and not a hallucinogenic substance?

**A.** Vertical or horizontal nystagmus
**B.** Pupillary dilation
**C.** Sweating
**D.** Tachycardia

**74** L. remains agitated and begins experiencing muscle spasms. The physician determines that he ingested phencyclidine. Which medication is most appropriate?

**A.** Diazepam (Valium)
**B.** Chlorpromazine (Thorazine)
**C.** Chlordiazepoxide (Librium)
**D.** Thiopental sodium (Pentothal)

---

### SITUATION

*N., a 30-year-old investment banker, voluntarily comes to the hospital for treatment of cocaine abuse. She has spent all of her savings and is heavily in debt to support a $500-a-day cocaine habit.*

*Questions 75 to 78 refer to this situation.*

**75** Which assessment finding indicates chronic cocaine use?

**A.** Craving for sweets
**B.** Lack of coordination
**C.** Pinpoint pupils
**D.** Nasal septum deterioration

**76** N.'s withdrawal from cocaine will most likely be evidenced by:

**A.** Depression and a strong craving for the drug
**B.** Restlessness and hallucinations
**C.** Seizures and tremors
**D.** Abdominal cramps and diaphoresis

**77** Which medication will the physician most likely prescribe for N. as she withdraws from cocaine?

**A.** Fluphenazine decanoate (Prolixin Decanoate)
**B.** Imipramine hydrochloride (Tofranil)
**C.** Phenelzine sulfate (Nardil)
**D.** Benztropine mesylate (Cogentin)

**78** Soon after N. is admitted to the detoxification unit, the nurse observes her scratching and clawing at her skin. This behavior is a sign of:

**A.** Allergy
**B.** Anxiety
**C.** Delusion
**D.** Hallucination

## SITUATION

*G., age 28, is the ex-wife of an intravenous drug abuser who died of acquired immunodeficiency syndrome (AIDS) 1 year ago. She has just been told that she has AIDS and is devastated by the news. G. recently started dating again and felt as though she was getting her life together after a disastrous marriage. She is being managed on an outpatient basis.*

*Questions 79 to 82 refer to this situation.*

**79** G. says to the nurse, "Why am I being punished for my husband's sins? How can God be so unjust?" Which response is most therapeutic?

**A.** "I have often asked the same question. There are so many innocent victims of AIDS. It isn't fair"
**B.** "Perhaps a clergyman can help you understand what is happening to you. Would you like me to arrange that?"
**C.** "Looking at this as punishment is a negative attitude. A positive outlook can help you fight this"
**D.** "It does seem unfair. You must be experiencing many strong emotions at this time. What are they?"

**80** G. expresses concern about her relationship with her new boyfriend. She tells the nurse that they have not yet had sexual intercourse and wonders whether she should tell him about her diagnosis before things progress to that level. The most appropriate initial response by the nurse is to:

**A.** Encourage G. to be completely honest with her boyfriend because he is at high risk for AIDS
**B.** Help G. consider the pros and cons of revealing her diagnosis at this time
**C.** Review ways to reduce her boyfriend's risk of contracting AIDS
**D.** Explain that disclosing her diagnosis is not an urgent matter because she is not yet acutely ill

**81** G. is admitted to the hospital for toxoplasmosis. Although she lives at home with her parents, she has not told them that she has AIDS. G.'s mother asks the nurse, "What is wrong with my daughter?" Which response is best?

**A.** "You'll have to ask your daughter. I cannot discuss her diagnosis with you"
**B.** "What has your daughter told you about her illness?"
**C.** "Your daughter is seriously ill and will need your love and support"
**D.** "Do you have any thoughts about what your daughter's diagnosis may be?"

**82** G. confides to the nurse that she is afraid to tell her parents she has AIDS because it would hurt them too much to know she is going to die. What is the most therapeutic response?

**A.** "Everyone is going to die at some time. What makes this so difficult for you to talk about?"
**B.** "I don't think you are giving your parents a fair chance"
**C.** "How do you feel about keeping something so important from them?"
**D.** "It sounds like you've been struggling with this decision. What might be the positive outcome of telling them?"

---

## SITUATION

*W., age 36, is brought to the emergency department by police, who report that he threatened his parents with a knife and threw sev-*

*eral pieces of furniture from the window of the family's apartment. This is W.'s sixth psychiatric admission in the past 4 years. His medical diagnosis is chronic paranoid schizophrenia.*

*Questions 83 to 90 refer to this situation.*

**83** The admitting nurse who reviews W.'s medical history should pay particular attention to identifying:

A. Length of stay during previous hospitalizations
B. History of hallucinations
C. History of violent behavior
D. Previous psychiatric diagnoses

**84** When W. is brought to the psychiatric unit, he appears extremely agitated. He paces back and forth in the dayroom, pushing anything that is in his way rather than walking around it. He mumbles angrily to himself as he paces. Which nursing intervention is most appropriate initially?

A. Call other staff members to help restrain the patient
B. Tell the patient that if he does not calm down, he will be restrained
C. Tell the patient to go to his room
D. Give the patient space and observe him closely

**85** A nurse can attempt to diffuse a patient's impending violent behavior by:

A. Helping him identify and express his feelings of anxiety and anger
B. Involving him in a quiet activity to divert his attention
C. Leaving him alone until he can talk about his feelings
D. Placing him in seclusion

**86** W.'s behavior continues to escalate. The nurse determines that restraints are necessary and asks the physician to write an order. The nurse knows that safe and effective restraint of a violent patient requires:

A. The assistance of seven or eight male staff members
B. A well-coordinated plan of action
C. Quick action
D. Administration of a PRN medication

**87** When staff members approach W. to restrain him, he says, "Don't touch me. I'll go wherever you want, just don't touch me." At this point, the staff should:

A. Proceed with the restraint procedure because it is safer than having W. act out
B. Step back and observe whether W. is in control
C. Step back and tell W. to go to the seclusion room
D. Tell W. that he will not be touched and accompany him to the seclusion room

**88** W. has been under close observation in the seclusion room for 1½ hours. He now calmly requests to be allowed out. Which nursing action is most effective when releasing a patient from seclusion?

A. Allow the patient to leave the room, but remain at a safe distance to give him enough space
B. Allow the patient to leave the room after securing a verbal contract from him that he will not act out
C. Open the seclusion room door periodically, but keep the patient inside until his behavior indicates that he is in control
D. Have two staff members enter the seclusion room to assess the patient's behavior before allowing him to leave

**89** W. is receiving haloperidol (Haldol) 10 mg P.O. t.i.d. Which side effects are most common with this medication?

A. Sedation and cardiovascular effects
B. Extrapyramidal effects
C. Dizziness and orthostatic hypotension
D. Anticholinergic effects

**90** One afternoon, W. refuses his 1:00 p.m. dose of haloperidol. Despite encouragement from the nurse, he states, "I don't want to take this any more." The nurse should:

A. Administer the medication by injection, if ordered
B. Request an as-needed prescription of chlorpromazine
C. Remind the patient that refusing his medication is negative behavior
D. Record and report the patient's refusal and monitor his behavior closely

---

## SITUATION

*D., an 83-year-old widow, is transferred to a skilled-nursing home from a community hospital. She lived with her daughter and family until she became confused and fell down several stairs, fracturing her hip and several ribs. D.'s daughter has multiple health problems and feels incapable of managing her mother at home.*

*Questions 91 to 95 refer to this situation.*

---

**91** D. seems distressed and confused by the transfer from the hospital to the nursing home. She cries and calls out for her daughter. The nurse has already explained the move several times. What should be done next?

**A.** Leave D. alone in a quiet, dimly lit environment to encourage rest and relaxation

**B.** Call D.'s daughter and have her speak with her mother

**C.** Remain with D., listen attentively, and reassure her about her new surroundings

**D.** Have several staff members and a few patients introduce themselves to D. to help orient her to her new environment

---

**92** D.'s daughter visits the day after admission. D. cries and pleads with her to take her home, saying "I'm going to die here." The daughter asks the nurse for advice. How should the nurse reply?

**A.** "This is very difficult for both you and your mother. Is there any way you can care for her at home?"

**B.** "It must be frightening to hear your mother say she's going to die. What are you feeling right now?"

**C.** "Try not to feel guilty. Your mother needs care and you cannot manage her at home"

**D.** "Many patients respond this way at first. She'll calm down once she gets to know the staff, patients, and routine here"

**93** D.'s daughter calls her mother's primary nurse to say that she has decided not to visit for a week or so. She has diabetes and her physician advised her to take it easy for a while. Which response is most supportive?

**A.** "You've had a rough time these last few weeks. Don't worry about your mother, she'll be fine"
**B.** "I can understand your need for a break. Keep in touch with me"
**C.** "Why don't you come in and we can discuss whether this is the best way to handle this
**D.** "It has been a difficult time for you both. Call me at any time. I'll call to let you know how she's doing"

**94** When planning D.'s care with the nursing assistants, the nurse should stress the importance of:

**A.** Establishing a predictable routine
**B.** Providing protective restraints
**C.** Limiting D.'s decision making to avoid anxiety
**D.** Diverting D. if she begins reminiscing about her past

**95** Which statement should the nurse keep in mind when caring for an older patient like D.?

**A.** Short-term memory often is impaired
**B.** Long-term memory often is impaired
**C.** Negativism should be expected
**D.** Confusion should be expected

## SITUATION

*R., age 16, is admitted for surgery to repair a hernia. His admission history indicates that he has Tourette's syndrome.*

*Questions 96 to 98 refer to this situation.*

**96** Which finding is most characteristic of Tourette's syndrome?

**A.** Echolalia
**B.** Echopraxia
**C.** Dyslexia
**D.** Coprolalia

**97** Which medication would the nurse expect the patient to be taking to control his Tourette's symptoms?

**A.** Diazepam (Valium)
**B.** Haloperidol (Haldol)
**C.** Amantadine hydrochloride (Symmetrel)
**D.** Phenelzine sulfate (Nardil)

**98** One of the nursing assistants assigned to care for R. refuses to go into his room, saying "He's a vulgar, obnoxious boy who needs his mouth washed out with soap." How should the nurse respond to the assistant?

**A.** Remind her that it is her duty to treat each patient the same and not to judge them
**B.** Agree with her and assign an assistant who is not disturbed by foul language to care for R.
**C.** Ignore her statement and continue making assignments based on the patient's needs
**D.** Acknowledge that the assistant's feelings are valid and ask the other assistants how they handle R.'s outbursts

## SITUATION

*I., a 60-year-old newly diagnosed Type I (insulin-dependent) diabetic patient is admitted to the medical-surgical unit. He is scheduled to undergo amputation of his lower left leg, which is gangrenous, the next morning.*

*Questions 99 and 100 refer to this situation.*

**99** The nurse finds I. sitting on the edge of his bed crying about the imminent loss of his leg. How should the nurse respond to seeing him this way?

**A.** Leave the patient alone to work out his grief
**B.** Sit beside the patient in silence until he stops crying, then ask him to explain what he is feeling
**C.** Attempt to comfort the patient by putting an arm around him
**D.** Try to distract the patient by talking about an upcoming local sports event

**100** Three weeks after his amputation, I. is transferred to a rehabilitation center for physical and occupational therapy. The nurse reviews I.'s medication regimen with him and asks if he has any questions or comments. I. responds, "Why should I even bother taking the medication? Without my leg, I won't be able to lead a normal life anyway." How should the nurse respond?

**A.** "In many ways, you won't be able to lead a normal life. How do you feel about that?"
**B.** "Don't be silly. Losing your leg shouldn't affect how normal you are or feel"
**C.** "I can't believe how defeated you sound. Don't you realize how lucky you are to be alive?"
**D.** "We have a great rehabilitative team here. Even though you won't be normal, I'm sure you'll be feeling like your old self within a few weeks"

# Answer sheet

| | A B C D | | A B C D | | A B C D | | A B C D |
|---|---|---|---|---|---|---|---|
| 1 | ○○○○ | 31 | ○○○○ | 61 | ○○○○ | 91 | ○○○○ |
| 2 | ○○○○ | 32 | ○○○○ | 62 | ○○○○ | 92 | ○○○○ |
| 3 | ○○○○ | 33 | ○○○○ | 63 | ○○○○ | 93 | ○○○○ |
| 4 | ○○○○ | 34 | ○○○○ | 64 | ○○○○ | 94 | ○○○○ |
| 5 | ○○○○ | 35 | ○○○○ | 65 | ○○○○ | 95 | ○○○○ |
| 6 | ○○○○ | 36 | ○○○○ | 66 | ○○○○ | 96 | ○○○○ |
| 7 | ○○○○ | 37 | ○○○○ | 67 | ○○○○ | 97 | ○○○○ |
| 8 | ○○○○ | 38 | ○○○○ | 68 | ○○○○ | 98 | ○○○○ |
| 9 | ○○○○ | 39 | ○○○○ | 69 | ○○○○ | 99 | ○○○○ |
| 10 | ○○○○ | 40 | ○○○○ | 70 | ○○○○ | 100 | ○○○○ |
| 11 | ○○○○ | 41 | ○○○○ | 71 | ○○○○ | | |
| 12 | ○○○○ | 42 | ○○○○ | 72 | ○○○○ | | |
| 13 | ○○○○ | 43 | ○○○○ | 73 | ○○○○ | | |
| 14 | ○○○○ | 44 | ○○○○ | 74 | ○○○○ | | |
| 15 | ○○○○ | 45 | ○○○○ | 75 | ○○○○ | | |
| 16 | ○○○○ | 46 | ○○○○ | 76 | ○○○○ | | |
| 17 | ○○○○ | 47 | ○○○○ | 77 | ○○○○ | | |
| 18 | ○○○○ | 48 | ○○○○ | 78 | ○○○○ | | |
| 19 | ○○○○ | 49 | ○○○○ | 79 | ○○○○ | | |
| 20 | ○○○○ | 50 | ○○○○ | 80 | ○○○○ | | |
| 21 | ○○○○ | 51 | ○○○○ | 81 | ○○○○ | | |
| 22 | ○○○○ | 52 | ○○○○ | 82 | ○○○○ | | |
| 23 | ○○○○ | 53 | ○○○○ | 83 | ○○○○ | | |
| 24 | ○○○○ | 54 | ○○○○ | 84 | ○○○○ | | |
| 25 | ○○○○ | 55 | ○○○○ | 85 | ○○○○ | | |
| 26 | ○○○○ | 56 | ○○○○ | 86 | ○○○○ | | |
| 27 | ○○○○ | 57 | ○○○○ | 87 | ○○○○ | | |
| 28 | ○○○○ | 58 | ○○○○ | 88 | ○○○○ | | |
| 29 | ○○○○ | 59 | ○○○○ | 89 | ○○○○ | | |
| 30 | ○○○○ | 60 | ○○○○ | 90 | ○○○○ | | |

## Answers and rationales

**1** Correct answer—**B**

Nursing models of psychiatric care view the person as a holistic being with biological, psychological, and sociocultural needs. Nursing models focus on the person not only as an individual but also as a member of a family, group, or community. Behavioral responses are viewed as part of a health-illness continuum and do not focus solely on health or illness. Nursing models include psychosocial and psychobiological perspectives.

**2** Correct answer—**A**

Hildegarde Peplau developed the first systematic theoretical framework for psychiatric nursing during the early 1950s. Her model, which describes the therapeutic nurse-patient relationship as a step-by-step process directed toward helping patients achieve their full potential, still is the basis for psychiatric nursing today. Madeleine Leininger's contributions are primarily in the area of transcultural nursing. Her work emphasizes the need for nurses to assess and analyze behaviors in the context of a person's cultural background. Dorothea Orem's "Self-Care Model" focuses on assisting patients to better health and improved self-care. Martha Rogers's "Science of Unitary Man" views humans and their environment in constant interaction within a unitary energy field; interactions between the nurse and patient repattern and change each energy field.

**3** Correct answer—**C**

Observations are descriptions of behaviors, whereas inferences are interpretations of behaviors. The statement "The patient does not respond to requests by staff members to shower and attend to personal grooming" describes staff actions and the patient's reactions without judging or interpreting the behavior. The other statements reflect the nurse's inferences, which may or may not be accurate interpretations. The nurse can attempt to validate her inferences by comparing them with those of other staff members but must keep in mind that the staff members may share her biases. A better way to validate inferences is to list the behaviors on which the inferences are made, then discuss them with others.

**4** Correct answer—**D**

In a therapeutic nurse-patient relationship, the nurse uses her knowledge and skills to plan interactions that help the patient meet his needs and facilitate his growth. Through use of the nursing process, the nurse assists the patient in establishing goals and priorities; she does not establish them by herself or allow the patient to determine the direction of the interactions. In a social relationship, both parties derive benefits and attempt to meet each other's needs. In a professional (nurse-patient) relationship, the patient's needs are always primary.

**5** Correct answer—**C**

During the working phase, the nurse and the patient explore relevant stressors and promote development of the patient's insight by linking perceptions, thoughts, feelings, and actions. The nurse helps the patient master his anxieties, increase his independence, and develop his coping mechanisms. The preinteraction phase, which occurs before the nurse meets with the patient, is the stage during which the nurse reviews and attempts to resolve her own anxieties, dependency issues, and fears. The introductory, or orientation, phase focuses on the initial assessment and provides data for identifying the patient's problems and setting initial goals. The termination phase prepares the patient for separation and ending the therapeutic relationship by reviewing progress and exploring feelings about termination.

**6** Correct answer—**D**

The patient is using the defense mechanism of undoing—performance of an action that partially negates a previous action—as he tries to rescind the fight he had with his wife. Displacement is a defense mechanism with which a patient shifts his emotions or feelings about a person or object toward a neutral or less dangerous person or object (for example, a patient who is angry at his boss and yells at his wife instead is displacing his negative feelings). Rationalization involves offering a socially acceptable or apparently logical excuse to justify otherwise unacceptable feelings, behaviors, or motives (for example, a student who fails an examination because he did not study and then blames his failure on the teacher's inadequate coverage of material in class is rationalizing his failure). In projection, a patient denies his own thoughts or impulses and attributes them to another person (for example, a man who denies his sexual feelings for a particular woman yet accuses that woman of flirting with him is projecting his feelings).

## 7 Correct answer—B

Regression is a retreat in the face of stress to behaviors characteristic of earlier developmental levels. Hospitalization can be stressful to a young child and may lead to such regressive behavior as bottle feeding and bed wetting. Denial is the avoidance of disagreeable realities by ignoring or refusing to recognize them (for example, a man who refuses to admit that his wife has a drinking problem even though she is an alcoholic is avoiding reality). Repression is the involuntary exclusion from awareness of painful or conflicting thoughts, impulses, or memories (for example, a woman who was sexually abused as a child yet has no recollection of such abuse is repressing this unpleasant experience). Sublimation is the substitution of a socially approved behavior or goal for a socially unacceptable drive (for example, a physically aggressive teenager who becomes a star football player instead of picking fights with others is sublimating his aggression).

## 8 Correct answer—A

A. is exhibiting reaction formation—conscious attitudes and behavioral patterns that are the opposite of her true feelings. Identification is the process of assuming the thoughts, mannerisms, or tastes of another person (for example, learning to appreciate opera because an admired person attends operas). Compensation is a defense mechanism with which a patient consciously attempts to make up for a deficiency in self-image by emphasizing another feature that he regards as an asset (for example, a short man who uses his loud, resonant voice to compensate for his small stature). Denial is avoiding reality by ignoring or refusing to recognize it.

## 9 Correct answer—D

The patient is denying the seriousness of her illness and the restrictions on her diet. In splitting, a patient views people and situations as either all good or all bad (for example, a woman finds no fault with her unfaithful husband even though he continues to have affairs). Compensation is a defense mechanism in which a person makes up for a deficiency in his self-image by strongly emphasizing some other feature. Rationalization permits a person to offer socially acceptable excuses to justify otherwise unacceptable impulses, feelings, behaviors, or motives.

## 10 Correct answer—C

In this situation, the patient is projecting (attributing) his own impulses to his roommate because of his anxiety about his own homosexual feelings. Displacement is the shifting of emotions from one person or object to another, less dangerous person or object. Intellectualization—the use of excessive logic to avoid unpleasant feelings—is evident when a newly diagnosed diabetic patient can explain his illness in detail but cannot express his feelings about the life-style changes he must make to manage the disease. In identification, a person emulates an admired person by taking on that person's thoughts, mannerisms, or tastes.

## 11 Correct answer—B

The dexamethasone suppression test (DST) is a blood test to determine cortisol levels after administration of dexamethasone (Decadron), which usually suppresses cortisol blood levels. The DST has gained considerable attention in the mental health field as a diagnostic marker for endogenous depression, as well as for its implications for treatment and prognosis of the disorder. Most studies have found that 40% to 50% of patients with endogenous depression or major depression with melancholia do not have a suppressed late-afternoon blood level of cortisol after administration of dexamethasone. Tests of coagulation profile, protein uptake, theophylline level, and follicle-stimulating hormone and thyroid-stimulating hormone levels are not useful for diagnosing depression.

## 12 Correct answer—C

Alcoholic hallucinosis typically occurs within the first 48 hours after an alcoholic patient stops drinking and is characterized by auditory hallucinations, delusions, and clouding of consciousness. Tactile and visual hallucinations occur later and are associated with alcohol withdrawal delirium (formerly delirium tremens). Olfactory hallucinations are more commonly seen in psychotic patients than in alcoholic patients.

## 13 Correct answer—B

Alcoholics Anonymous (AA) is a worldwide organization of self-help groups for alcoholic persons who want to stop drinking. Groups of recovering alcoholics provide support and assistance to other alcoholic patients. Through meetings and sponsorship, alcoholic persons are helped to maintain their sobriety one day at a time. AA is not led by professionals, and its only focus is on helping alcoholics remain sober. Education and research are conducted by other groups, including the National Council on Alcoholism and the National Institute on Alcoholism and Alcohol Abuse.

## 14 Correct answer—D

The maximum daily dosage of thioridazine (Mellaril) is 800 mg; dosages exceeding this amount are associated with retinitis pigmentosa, an irreversible condition that can be avoided if dosage limits are observed. The recommended maintenance dosage range for thioridazine, an antipsychotic agent, is 300 to 800 mg/day. Recommended dosage ranges for chlorpromazine (Thorazine), an antipsychotic agent, and alprazolam (Xanax), an antianxiety agent, are 300 to 1,400 mg/day and 0.5 to 4 mg/day, respectively. Dosages for lithium (Lithane), an antimania drug, are usually individualized to achieve a maintenance blood level of 0.6 to 1.2 mEq/liter.

## 15 Correct answer—A

Neuroleptic malignant syndrome is a rare but life-threatening condition characterized by hyperthermia, tachycardia, muscular rigidity and tremor, stupor, incontinence, leukocytosis, elevated serum creatinine phosphokinase levels, hyperkalemia, renal failure, rapid pulse and respiratory rates, and diaphoresis. This syndrome can develop rapidly and is most common in young men who become dehydrated and are being treated with several antipsychotic medications, especially high-potency ones. Neuroleptic malignant syndrome is treated with supportive measures, such as hydration, dialysis, fever reduction, adequate ventilation, and discontinuance of all medications. Pseudoparkinsonism, sedation, and blurred vision are common but less serious side effects of antipsychotic drugs. They should be reported and treated with appropriate nursing and medical interventions.

## 16 Correct answer—B

Certain amino acids (tyrosine, phenylalanine, cysteine, and glutamic acid) are the precursors of neurotransmitters. These amino acids may be prescribed to replace the neurotransmitters depleted by cocaine abuse. Restoring neurotransmitter levels at the neuronal synapses alleviates the depression and fatigue caused by withdrawal from cocaine. Tricyclic antidepressants also may be used to restore neurotransmitters. Amino acids do not compensate for nutritional deficiencies, reduce agitation, or detoxify residual cocaine.

## 17 Correct answer—B

A patient taking monoamine oxidase (MAO) inhibitor antidepressants, such as tranylcypromine (Parnate), should not eat foods containing tyramine. Specifically, the patient should avoid consuming chicken livers, Chianti wine, beer, ale, aged game meats, broad beans, aged cheeses, sour cream, avocados, yogurt, pickled herring, yeast extract, chocolate, excessive caffeine, vanilla, and soy sauce. The patient also must refrain from taking cold and hay fever preparations that contain vasoconstrictors.

## 18 Correct answer—C

Most neuroleptic agents, such as chlorpromazine, induce anticholinergic side effects similar to those produced by atropine. Dry mouth, blurred vision, and stuffy nose are commonly experienced early in the course of treatment. Dry mouth can cause excessive fluid intake that results in excess fluid volume and electrolyte imbalances. The evidence is insufficient to formulate nursing diagnoses of *Urge incontinence related to excessive fluid intake, Impaired adjustment related to anxiety,* or *Fatigue related to continual pacing.*

## 19 Correct answer—B

Chewing sugarless gum promotes salivation and helps keep the buccal mucosa moist. Sucking on sour hard candy may achieve the same effect. Sugarless gum or candy should be offered because gum or candy with a high sugar content promotes dental caries. Forbidding fluid intake, taking B. to his room, and providing emotional support do not address the patient's immediate problem (dry mouth) and do not alleviate the cause of his excess fluid intake.

## 20 Correct answer—C

Asking the patient to discuss his brother indicates a willingness to listen. As the patient talks, the nurse can help him address painful feelings by offering support and can strengthen the nurse-patient relationship by demonstrating empathy. A strong nurse-patient relationship is the best deterrent to suicide because suicidal persons typically feel alone and isolated. Encouraging the patient to talk about his brother and his feelings also enables the nurse to assess whether suicide precautions are necessary at this time. Instead of denying or arguing about the reality of the patient's hallucinations, the nurse should focus on issues that are based in reality.

## 21 Correct answer—D

B.'s behavior suggests that he may be dizzy. Dizziness when changing from a lying or sitting position to a standing position indicates orthostatic hypotension, a side effect associated with antipychotic drugs, such as chlorpromazine. The nurse should assess the patient's blood pressure immediately while he is sitting or lying and again while he is standing. Orthostatic hypotension is marked by a diastolic difference of 40 mm Hg. Observing the patient from a distance, reorienting him, and encouraging him to stay in his room provide no information about his condition.

## 22 Correct answer—A

The nurse should teach a patient with orthostatic hypotension to rise slowly to prevent abrupt drops in blood pressure associated with positional change. Providing one-to-one supervision, having the patient remain in bed, and paging the physician may ensure B.'s safety but do not encourage him to cope with dizziness.

## 23 Correct answer—C

Extrapyramidal signs, which are a common side effect of neuroleptic medications, are similar to those of a person with Parkinson's disease. They include muscle rigidity, pill-rolling tremor (rubbing the fingers together as if rolling dough into balls), masklike facies (facial muscle rigidity), propulsive gait, and drooling. Extrapyramidal side effects are not dose related.

## 24 Correct answer—A

Extrapyramidal signs, sometimes called pseudoparkinsonism, can be relieved by administering medications used to treat Parkinson's disease, such as trihexyphenidyl (Artane), procyclidine (Kemadrin), and benztropine mesylate (Cogentin). The nurse must confer with the physician to obtain a written order for the addition of antiparkinson medication to B.'s therapeutic regimen. Relaxation techniques and reassurance will not relieve the extrapyramidal signs. The nurse should not withhold the next dose of medication because this action would not relieve the signs and might increase the psychotic behavior.

## 25 Correct answer—D

The patient should be instructed to avoid driving a car and operating machinery while taking neuroleptic medications because these drugs can cause drowsiness, tremors, and blurred vision, placing him at high risk for injury. Staying away from persons with upper respiratory tract infections or spending time outdoors is good advice but not critical. The use of neuroleptic agents does not require dietary restrictions.

## 26 Correct answer—B

Some neuroleptic agents, including chlorpromazine, cause extreme sensitivity to sunlight, which can result in severe sunburn with even minimal exposure to ultraviolet light. The nurse should advise the patient to use a potent sunscreen or sun-blocking lotion whenever exposure to the sun is likely. A ski mask would be only minimally helpful. Neither knowing B.'s whereabouts nor having him take vitamin D will prevent him from becoming sunburned.

## 27 Correct answer—B

Because neuroleptic drugs enhance alcohol's central nervous system depressant effect, the patient taking a neuroleptic medication should understand that drinking alcoholic beverages is dangerous. He also should avoid taking over-the-counter medication and recreational drugs because the potential for unexpected interactions is high. He should limit his coffee and tea intake because of their stimulant effect. Cathartics usually are not contraindicated for a patient taking neuroleptic medication. Neuroleptic medications do not cause allergic reactions to antibiotics.

## 28 Correct answer—D

A mental status examination of a depressed patient includes a careful assessment of her mood (affect). Besides sadness, other characteristic affects of a depressed person include irritability, apathy, self-doubt, agitation, hostility, anger, lethargy, shame, and lack of pleasure in things that normally give pleasure (anhedonia). Self-blame and low self-esteem also may be present. A depressed patient may be emotionally labile, crying easily one moment and laughing the next.

## 29 Correct answer—B

MAO inhibitors, such as phenelzine sulfate (Nardil), do not need to be taken 1 hour before meals. However, any patient taking such drugs must be aware of certain dietary precautions. For example, the patient must avoid foods containing tyramine—aged cheeses, sour cream, beer, red wine (especially Chianti), yogurt, yeasts, pickled herring, aged meats, meat tenderizers, and chicken livers—because of the possibility of hypertensive reactions. The patient can drink small amounts of white wine because this type of wine does not undergo the prolonged aging that results in tyramine formation. The patient also should limit her intake of chocolate and caffeine because these substances have been reported to cause blood pressure elevations in persons taking MAO inhibitors. The nurse should instruct the patient to report any early signs of an impending hypertensive reaction (headache, palpitations, neck stiffness, sweating, nausea, and photophobia). Because MAO inhibitors can cause drowsiness, the patient should take extra care when driving or avoid driving if this is possible.

## 30 Correct answer—C

The nurse can best help S. to cope with her feelings by encouraging her to discuss her loss while offering comfort and support. Loss of a significant relationship through death or divorce may lead to depression if the person who experiences the loss cannot resolve her grief. Telling the patient to forget the past is inappropriate and can promote unresolved grief. Group therapy would be helpful only after S. has worked with the nurse on issues related to her loss. Platitudes, such as "time heals all wounds" only devalue the patient's feelings.

## 31 Correct answer—A

Nursing interventions for a depressed patient include education and support related to the grieving process. The nurse must assure the patient that she will not cry forever, lose control, or go crazy if she expresses her grief. On the contrary, such events may occur if the patient does not grieve. Reflecting back what the patient has said does not provide the information she needs to understand her experience or the emotional support she needs to express her feelings. Additional medication is not the answer because it relieves only the symptoms, not the underlying cause. Until Mrs. S. can express her emotions and experience her grief, her guilt feelings probably will not subside.

## 32 Correct answer—B

It is unusual for a 6-month-old infant to be indifferent to the actions of strangers in his environment. Infants at this age usually begin to show fear of strangers and are inquisitive, interested in their surroundings, and constantly in motion. Indifference to others may be an indication of autism. The nurse expects the infant to respond to his name unless he is hearing impaired. Reaching for the stethoscope and fidgeting when held are normal responses for a 6-month-old infant.

## 33 Correct answer—C

Autistic children operate from their own reality. They typically are withdrawn and mute, and they display a lack of anticipatory response to being picked up. Normal growth and development of a 6-month-old infant includes increased verbal skills, verbal and nonverbal demands to be picked up, and increased environmental awareness.

## 34 Correct answer—A

Early indications of deviant social development include the child's lack of emotional response to his parents, limpness or stiffening when being held, and absent or extremely limited babbling and other forms of nonverbal communication. Early signs of autism include nonresponsiveness to people and preoccupation with inanimate objects. A healthy 6-month-old infant who is uncomfortable or seeks attention may cry frequently or want to be held constantly. It is normal for a child of this age to prefer one person to another.

## 35 Correct answer—B

Evidence suggests that a combination of behavior modification, chemotherapy, psychotherapy, and milieu therapy may decrease the maladaptive behaviors in a child with deviant social development if the interventions are undertaken before the behaviors are firmly entrenched. It is unlikely that early treatment will cure autism. Because autistic children do not respond to cuddling, teaching the mother how to cuddle properly is inappropriate. Expecting an autistic infant to become spontaneous and responsive is unrealistic.

## 36 Correct answer—B

The physician probably will prescribe imipramine (Tofranil), a tricyclic antidepressant commonly used to treat depression.
Lorazepam (Ativan) and alprazolam (Xanax) are used to treat anxiety. Thiothixene (Navane) is an antipsychotic medication.

## 37 Correct answer—D

The patient can expect a full therapeutic response to her tricyclic antidepressant medication in about 3 to 4 weeks. However, after 7 to 10 days, she should begin noticing improvements in her sleep and appetite and possibly her mood. The nurse should offer reassurance during this time because the patient may expect a quicker recovery and be frustrated by the slow progress.

## 38 Correct answer—B

The exact mechanism of action of electroconvulsive therapy (ECT) is unknown, although various theories exist. One theory, which is not widely accepted among medical authorities, suggests that a depressed patient's underlying guilt feelings are relieved by his perception of ECT as a punishment. Another hypothesis suggests that ECT increases the levels of chemicals in the brain, such as the neurotransmitters acetylcholine, norepinephrine, and serotonin. Although authorities agree that ECT does not result in any permanent brain damage, they do not necessarily recognize a connection between increased chemical levels in the brain and ECT. No similarity between the action of ECT and that of antidepressant medication has been proven.

## 39 Correct answer—D

Before B. undergoes ECT, the nurse should ensure that the patient's lithium therapy has been discontinued because lithium prolongs the effects of succinylcholine chloride, a muscle relaxant that is given just before the shock. The nurse also must ensure that the patient has had a medical evaluation that includes an electrocardiogram, a chest X-ray, neurologic and laboratory tests, and spinal X-rays, if indicated. The patient's chart should contain a signed informed consent as well as documentation that the patient and her family have been taught about the procedure and what to expect afterward.

## 40 Correct answer—C

A patient undergoing ECT should be prepared in a manner similar to that for general anesthesia. For example, the patient should receive nothing by mouth for 8 hours before the procedure to reduce the likelihood of vomiting and aspiration; she should void before treatment to decrease the possibility of involuntary voiding during the procedure; she should remove any full dentures, glasses, or jewelry to prevent breakage or loss; and she should wear a hospital gown or loose-fitting clothing to allow unrestricted movement. These preparations are not usually indicated for a patient undergoing physical therapy, neurologic examination, or cardiac stress testing.

## 41 Correct answer—D

A patient undergoing ECT can expect to experience certain adverse effects as a result of treatment; backache, however, is not among them. Part of the nurse's responsibility is to prepare the patient for expected effects and to offer support and comfort should they occur. During the course of treatment, which may last for several sessions, the patient probably will have short- and long-term memory impairment; the nurse should reassure the patient that this will subside gradually after the therapy has ended. Upon awakening after each treatment session, the patient most likely will be confused; the nurse should reorient her to person, place, and time. The patient also may have a headache after each session, so the nurse should be prepared to administer an analgesic, as ordered.

## 42 Correct answer—D

When a nurse encounters a patient who appears to be hallucinating, she must recognize that the patient has impaired perception and communication ability. Speaking to such a patient in simple, concrete terms helps him to focus on reality. A hallucinating patient also may be confused, disoriented, and frightened, so the nurse must help him to understand his surroundings through reality orientation. Failing to acknowledge the patient's disorientation by remaining silent or treating him as if he were normal, or allowing the patient to verbalize freely while hallucinating, is not therapeutic.

## 43 Correct answer—A

When responding to an hallucinating patient, the nurse must first orient him to reality. Telling C. that she understands that the voices are real to him but that she does not hear them provides reality testing without denying the patient's experience. Having established reality orientation, the nurse can assess the content of the voices. Offering reassurances that nothing will happen or that many patients hear voices is unlikely to be effective.

## 44 Correct answer—B

Photosensitivity and parkinsonian tremors are common side effects of phenothiazines, such as trifluoperazine (Stelazine). Diazepam (Valium) and oxazepam (Serax) are benzodiazepine-derivative antianxiety agents; meprobamate (Miltown) is a carbamate-derivative antianxiety agent. Common adverse effects of these antianxiety drugs include dizziness, drowsiness, and ataxia.

## 45 Correct answer—B

The nurse should focus on reality and avoid reinforcing the patient's hallucinations by responding positively to the patient's discussion of them. Interventions should be directed at identifying the needs met by the hallucinations and acting to meet those needs more appropriately. The nurse also should provide positive feedback to the patient when he faces reality and should try to prevent his retreat into fantasy.

## 46 Correct answer—C

Although a schizophrenic patient may display delusions of grandeur (behaving as if he has extraordinary powers or is highly important), C. is not displaying any behavior to reflect this condition. Many schizophrenic patients have difficulty with gender identity and sexuality, which results in fear and anxiety. Projecting these feelings onto others is a defense mechanism commonly used by schizophrenic patients.

## 47 Correct answer—**D**

Assigning C. to a private room will best decrease his anxiety by removing him from what he perceives to be a threatening situation. Increasing the dosage of the patient's medication is a medical, not nursing, intervention. Restricting C. to his room for extended periods is inappropriate unless he is so agitated that he may lose control. Besides, separating C. from others by restricting him to his room may increase his anxiety and paranoia. Confronting C. about his feelings may be too threatening to be effective and probably would only increase his defensiveness.

## 48 Correct answer—**B**

The most therapeutic response is for the nurse to reassure the patient that she is interested in him and his welfare. Confronting the patient about his suspiciousness at such an early point in the nurse-patient relationship is threatening and nontherapeutic, as is questioning the patient further about his suspicions. Because a suspicious patient thinks rigidly, he probably will not accept a rational argument that the nurse has never met his wife or boss before.

## 49 Correct answer—**C**

When responding to a suspicious, delusional patient, the nurse must clearly present the reality of the situation without lending credence to or challenging the patient's perceptions. Since improving the patient's reality testing is a goal with suspicious patients, ignoring J.'s remark by offering to take him for a walk misses an opportunity for therapeutic intervention. Delving further into the delusion and offering to protect the patient confirm his perception and do not improve his reality testing.

## 50 Correct answer—**D**

Providing J. with packaged, high-protein between-meal snacks will help him maintain his nutritional status until he feels safe enough to eat his meals. The patient's suspicions may be reinforced if the nurse focuses on his eating or inquires about what is wrong with his meal. Although allowing J. to continue to observe his tablemates is appropriate, it does not help him meet his nutritional needs. Accepting the patient's behavior while providing him with alternative nutrition is the most effective approach.

## 51 Correct answer—C

Providing a suspicious patient with an activity that requires a high level of concentration helps keep the patient focused on reality and allows less time for delusional thinking. Such a patient tends to prefer projects that require attention to detail, such as painting by numbers, to help relieve anxiety. Challenging a suspicious patient with various tasks will not help keep him focused on reality. A suspicious patient tends to maintain interest in projects even if not concentrating at a high level. Physically acting out is not typical of a suspicious patient.

## 52 Correct answer—A

Attention deficit disorder (ADD) is a type of learning disability characterized by impulsivity and inattentiveness, which result in the child's inability to achieve his full academic potential despite having an average to above-average intelligence. Below-average intelligence and marked deficits in adaptive behavior are signs of mental retardation. An overt lack of regard for authority and the rights of others is characteristic of conduct disorder. A child with ADD usually has no signs of impaired thinking or emotional instability.

## 53 Correct answer—B

*Potential for injury related to impulsivity* is the only applicable nursing diagnosis at this time. Because of D.'s inability to sit still and his tendency to react impulsively and engage in fighting, the nurse must develop an effective plan to protect him and others from injury. The other diagnoses either do not address the child's needs or fail to reflect the actual situation. The history findings do not offer any evidence of ineffective family coping, mutism, or impaired thinking.

## 54 Correct answer—C

Cerebral stimulants, such as methylphenidate (Ritalin) and dextro-amphetamine sulfate (Dexedrine), are the drugs of choice for treating ADD. These agents have a paradoxic (opposite) effect on children and have been used successfully to increase attention span. Antipsychotic agents, such as chlorpromazine (Thorazine), and antidepressants, such as impiramine (Tofranil), are sometimes ordered in addition to central nervous stimulants for children who have ADD with hyperactivity. Sedatives and antianxiety agents generally are not used to treat ADD.

## 55  Correct answer—**D**

Delayed physical growth resulting from the use of cerebral stimulants commonly is the greatest concern of parents who have children with ADD. The nurse must assure the parents that the drug's effects on growth are minor and that growth resumes once the dosage is decreased. Although dizziness, headache, and increased appetite may occur with use of cerebral stimulants, such side effects usually are of a lesser concern to parents.

## 56  Correct answer—**C**

J.'s history indicates a conduct disorder—a repetitive pattern of behavior in which a person disregards or violates the rights of others. A child with conduct disorder cannot delay self-gratification and may have had little experience with limit setting. Therefore, a consistent, firm, and nonpunitive approach is best. Passive friendliness—remaining supportive and accessible to the patient without seeking to interact with him—is an approach primarily used by nurses working with paranoid patients. Active friendliness—actively seeking interaction with the patient—is useful for depressed patients. Laissez-faire—interacting at will with no specific goals in mind—is useful in community meetings involving both staff members and patients. This approach is not therapeutic for a patient with conduct disorder because he needs a more structured and consistent pattern of interaction.

## 57  Correct answer—**D**

Therapeutic communication aims to recognize the patient's feelings and encourage further elaboration. The nurse's telling the patient that she understands "things haven't been easy..." demonstrates empathy and promotes discussion. Responses that impose the nurse's judgment ("Your brother should be more important to you than your friends"), negate the patient's feelings ("Are you afraid we'll find something wrong with you also?"), or belittle her feelings ("Don't be silly"), are nontherapeutic and can hinder communication and the nurse's ability to help.

## 58 Correct answer—**B**

A patient with conduct disorder of the unsocialized aggressive type tends to strike out at others; therefore, a primary goal is to decrease the patient's hostility and aggression toward others. Such a patient lacks the emotional depth needed to sustain interpersonal relationships with anyone, including family members and friends, so his behavior is unlikely to be influenced by peers. Because the patient exhibits little guilt over his behavior, fostering a sense of accountability for his actions would be futile. A child with this diagnosis does not typically engage in self-mutilating behavior.

## 59 Correct answer—**C**

Antisocial personality disorder, a pervasive general disregard for others, is characterized by selfishness, manipulation, and egocentrism. Although onset usually is before age 15, the disorder is not diagnosed before age 18 because an extended period is needed to document consistent patterns of antisocial behavior. Also, clinicians are hesistant to label a child as antisocial. Borderline personality disorder is evidenced by emotional lability, unpredictability, and impulsiveness. Schizoid personality disorder is characterized by withdrawal, seclusion, coldness, and aloofness. Passive-aggressive personality disorder is marked by intentional inefficiency, procrastination, and dawdling.

## 60 Correct answer—**D**

Because ensuring the safety of the patient and the nurse is the priority at this time, the nurse should cautiously approach M. while calling her name and talking to her in a calm, confident manner. The nurse should keep in mind that the patient must not be startled or overwhelmed; she should explain in simple terms that she is there to help, then carefully observe the patient's response. If the patient shows signs of agitation or confusion or poses a threat, the nurse should retreat and request assistance. The nurse should not attempt to sit next to the patient or examine her injuries without first announcing her presence and assessing the dangers of the situation.

## 61 Correct answer—**C**

Most states provide for some type of emergency admission for patients who pose an immediate threat to themselves or others. Typically, the time of commitment ranges from 3 to 30 days, and the patient can request an examination by a physician of her own choosing. By explaining the consequences of the emergency admission and informing the patient of her right to see a lawyer, the nurse is acting to protect the patient's rights. A patient has rights in all admission situations, and the nurse has a responsibility to give the patient clear information about these rights and ensure that they are not violated. Telling the patient that she has no right to leave without explaining why is inappropriate. Agreeing with the patient that she was stupid to cut her wrists will alienate her and hinder the establishment of a therapeutic relationship. Acknowledging that the patient is upset is helpful, but giving false reassurance that she may be released sooner is not.

## 62 Correct answer—B

A patient's suicide plan is considered the most significant criterion for determining suicide potential. A patient who describes a specific plan (what she will do, when, and how), has access to the means, and has a highly lethal plan in mind (gunshot, jumping, or hanging versus overdosing or wrist slashing) is considered at high risk for suicide. Although the nurse should assess all factors—including previous suicide attempts, emotional state, and self-esteem—during a comprehensive mental status examination, she should view the suicide plan as the most significant determinant. Although M.'s wrist slashing is considered less lethal than gunshot, jumping, or hanging, it should be reported and treated seriously, as should all suicidal threats, gestures, and attempts.

## 63 Correct answer—D

Despite her discomfort over a lack of privacy, the patient requires constant observation. This means that a nurse must remain with her at all times, even when she is using the bathroom. Empathizing with the patient ("I would probably feel uncomfortable, too...") acknowledges the legitimacy of the patient's feelings. Clearly stating the rationale for the nurse's actions ("ensuring your safety is my first priority...") reassures the patient that her safety will be protected. The nurse should not judge the patient's behavior or apologize for her presence. Agreeing to leave the patient alone for even a brief period displays poor judgment and may endanger the patient.

## 64 Correct answer—A

The priority goal in this situation is to have M. identify available support systems to help with managing stress while an outpatient. Since the problems leading to M.'s suicide attempt probably have not been resolved during her 5-day hospitalization, the nurse must help her to establish a reliable support network to help her cope with any expected or unexpected stressors. The nurse can best assist M. by providing names and phone numbers of outpatient personnel and contacting the outpatient therapist before discharge. She also should provide her with phone numbers of suicide prevention hotlines and community help centers. Encouraging M. to express shame or guilt is nontherapeutic and likely to exacerbate the suicidal crisis. Premature elevation of mood in a suicidal patient should be regarded with caution because a patient who has made up her mind about a new suicide plan or is just emerging from a deep depression typically has more energy to act upon her suicidal ideas. Although M. may have been only seeking attention by slashing her wrists, the nurse should not minimize the significance of the suicide attempt.

## 65 Correct answer—C

The nurse should approach A. calmly, sit down with him, and have him attempt to focus on a few essential questions. The nurse needs to assess the patient's level of reality testing, his understanding of the reason for admission, and his mental status to establish preliminary nursing diagnoses and plan related nursing interventions. Trying to make the patient sit quietly while completing the interview would prove frustrating for the patient and the nurse. Walking around with him would be too stimulating and anxiety-provoking for both parties. Postponing the initial interview is unrealistic; the information and observations obtained from such an interview are necessary to determine the patient's mental status and to plan appropriate initial interventions.

## 66 Correct answer—A

The nurse should withhold administering the lithium until she has had a chance to question the physician about the prescription. Administering lithium 600 mg P.O. stat is inappropriate because lithium has no sedative effects and does not reach a therapeutic blood level (1 to 1.5 mEq/liter) for 7 to 14 days. Also, because lithium is excreted by the kidneys and can cause some thyroid dysfunction, the patient should not begin lithium therapy until he has undergone a complete history and physical examination, including a thorough evaluation of kidney and thyroid function. Asking the physician to prescribe chlorpromazine (Thorazine) as needed is appropriate only if the patient becomes uncontrollable. To help manage the hyperactivity of an acute manic episode, an antipsychotic (not antiparkinsonian) medication usually is administered before and during lithium therapy until therapeutic blood levels of lithium are attained.

## 67 Correct answer—A

Although A. should be encouraged to eat a regular diet without supplements, the best intervention at this time is to monitor his intake, output, and weight on a daily basis. These measurements allow the nurse to assess the patient's nutritional needs. Even though A. is still 15 lb overweight, a weight loss of 20 lb in 1 month is drastic. If the nurse notices that the patient is not eating or is eating poorly, she can offer supplements in the form of finger foods and high-protein drinks to provide proper nutrition. Because a manic patient typically expends much energy on activity and does not allow for sufficient rest and proper nutrition, promoting exercise is not recommended.

## 68 Correct answer—D

Setting limits is essential for an acutely manic patient. When the nurse observes any escalation in the patient's behavior, she should speak to the patient matter-of-factly and accompany him to a quieter, less stimulating environment, such as his room. Ignoring A.'s hyperactivity and manipulation of other patients would be inappropriate because such disruptive behavior may result in a dangerous situation. Confronting A. in front of the other patients also is inappropriate because the nurse must do her best to maintain the patient's self-esteem. Limit-setting interventions for a new patient are best handled by staff members. Until A. has adjusted to his environment and feels less threatened, the nurse should not encourage other patients to confront him about his behavior.

## 69 Correct answer—D

A manic patient with a sleep pattern disturbance requires special interventions to promote adequate rest and prevent exhaustion. Permitting A. to interact with a staff member when he cannot sleep does not promote the rest he needs; rather, it draws attention to the patient's not sleeping and implies that staying awake is acceptable as long as he is talking with a staff member. Offering a prescribed sedative can enhance the patient's ability to get needed rest. Daytime naps are helpful but should be limited so that they do not interfere with sleeping at night. Teaching A. relaxation techniques is an excellent way of promoting comfort and reducing stimuli so that he can rest.

## 70 Correct answer—A

A manic patient needs assistance in recognizing and expressing his emotions. By reflecting back A.'s anger, the nurse helps him to identify his emotion and acknowledges that anger is an appropriate reaction in this situation. Encouraging A. to tell P. what he would like him to do the next time he wants to borrow something provides the patient with an acceptable forum for expressing what he is feeling. Acknowledging A.'s feelings without helping him to express his concerns is less helpful. Telling A. that he is losing control and making no sense fails to acknowledge the patient's feelings and demonstrates a lack of empathy on the part of the nurse. By sending A. to his room without exploring his feelings, the nurse fails to take advantage of an opportunity to enhance the patient's understanding and expression of emotion.

## 71 Correct answer—C

The nurse should instruct A. to take his 1:00 p.m. dose of lithium now and his next dose, as scheduled, at 5:00 p.m. If a patient misses the dosing time by more than 2 hours, the nurse should instruct him to skip that dose and take the regular dose at the next scheduled time. A patient should never be told to double the dose to make up for missed medication, because lithium blood levels peak about 3 hours after administration and doubling a dose can produce toxic effects. Rescheduling the patient's doses would be confusing and could lead to further dosing errors.

## 72 Correct answer—D

Maintaining the safety of the patient and others in the emergency department should be the primary focus of care. Acute toxic psychosis can result from the ingestion of hallucinogenic drugs or phencyclidine (PCP). A patient under the influence of either of these drugs may experience perceptual distortions and panic and act out impulsively, thus posing a threat to himself and others. Hallucinogens do not cause withdrawal symptoms. Sedating the patient is not recommended until the ingested substance has been positively identified. Waiting for the drug's effect to wear off is inappropriate; the patient may exhibit psychotic behavior and flashbacks for some time and should be watched closely to maintain safety. Persons who have used hallucinogens have been known to jump from windows and display other dangerous behavior associated with the perceptual disturbances caused by drug use.

## 73 Correct answer—A

Within an hour after ingesting PCP, a patient may experience two or more of the following symptoms: vertical or horizontal nystagmus, increased blood pressure and heart rate, diminished pain response, ataxia, and dysarthria. Ingestion of hallucinogenics is followed by at least two of the following symptoms: pupillary dilation, sweating, tachycardia, palpitations, tremors, blurred vision, and incoordination. Both types of drugs cause altered behavior, including perceptual disturbances, impaired judgment, and delusions.

## 74 Correct answer—A

Diazepam (Valium), an anxiolytic anticonvulsant, can relieve the muscle spasms and agitation associated with phencyclidine ingestion. Chlordiazepoxide (Librium) is less effective in controlling these symptoms. Chlorpromazine (Thorazine), an anticholinergic, would not be used because phencyclidine also has anticholinergic properties; the interaction of these two drugs would exacerbate the anticholinergic effects, resulting in urine retention, dry mouth, decreased sweating, and constipation. Thiopental sodium (Pentothal), a short-acting barbiturate, is not used to control behavior, nor is it used as a long-term muscle relaxant.

## 75 Correct answer—D

Chronic inhalation of cocaine produces burns, sores, and deterioration of the nasal membranes and nasal septum. Characteristic signs of cocaine abuse include a chronic runny nose, nasal irritation, and repeated wiping and rubbing of the nose. Abusers of marijuana, hashish, and tetrahydrocannabinal (THC) typically crave sweets. Abusers of barbiturates, sedatives, or hypnotics commonly show a lack of coordination when intoxicated. Pinpoint pupils are evident after abuse of opiates, such as heroin and morphine, and opioids, such as methadone; dilated pupils are noted during withdrawal from these drugs.

## 76 Correct answer—A

Cocaine withdrawal symptoms include extreme depression ("post-coke blues") and severe craving for the drug, as well as anxiety, fatigue, and insomnia. Cocaine abuse causes a strong psychological dependence on the drug; physical addiction to the drug has not yet been clearly established. Restlessness and hallucinations are symptoms of cocaine overdose. Tremors and occasionally seizures are common in patients withdrawing from barbiturates. Withdrawal from opiates is marked by abdominal cramping and diaphoresis.

## 77 Correct answer—B

The physician will probably prescribe imipramine hydrochloride (Tofranil), a tricyclic antidepressant, for several weeks to combat the depression associated with detoxification and withdrawal from cocaine. Tricyclic antidepressants increase the neurotransmitter levels at the neural synapses that have been depleted by cocaine abuse. Fluphenazine decanoate (Prolixin Decanoate) is a long-acting antipsychotic medication used primarily for maintenance therapy. Its slow onset of action (24 to 72 hours) and long duration of effect (4 weeks) make it unsuitable for patients withdrawing from cocaine. Phenelzine sulfate (Nardil), a monoamine oxidase inhibitor antidepressant with many contraindications and potential interactions with other drugs and foods, would not be the first choice for a cocaine abuser. Benztropine mesylate (Cogentin) is used to treat drug-induced extrapyramidal symptoms.

## 78 Correct answer—D

A patient who has ingested large amounts of cocaine may experience tactile hallucinations. Such a patient typically reports feeling bugs crawling under her skin and scratches vigorously in an attempt to rid herself of this sensation. Haloperidol (Haldol) is used to control these symptoms. The sensation of bugs crawling under the skin is an altered perception, not an allergic reaction, a sign of anxiety, or a delusion (altered thinking).

## 79 Correct answer—D

G.'s response to her diagnosis is typical of that of patients with serious and life-threatening illnesses—she is angry and resents the unfairness of her situation. When responding to the patient, the nurse should acknowledge that G.'s feelings are normal and help her ventilate her anger. For the nurse to indicate that she has the same questions as the patient would only reinforce the patient's perception that her illness is a punishment from God. Talking with a clergyman can help, but offering to call the clergy so quickly implies that the nurse is unwilling to listen to the patient. Although the nurse should foster a positive outlook, telling G. to have a positive attitude cuts her off and suggests that the nurse is unwilling to address her intimate disclosures.

## 80 Correct answer—B

The patient should decide for herself whether or not to reveal her diagnosis of acquired immunodeficiency syndrome (AIDS) to her boyfriend; however, the nurse can help her to explore the pros and cons of disclosing this information to him and others before making a decision. The nurse must consider what is best for the patient and help her to see how disclosing her diagnosis at this time might positively or negatively affect her ensuing relationship and the level of intimacy she hopes to achieve.

Although G.'s boyfriend is at low risk for AIDS (they have not yet engaged in sexual intercourse), the nurse must provide G. with information on safe sex practices and ways to reduce the risk of transmitting AIDS. Such a discussion, although important, should be secondary to the immediate one involving G.'s decision to disclose her diagnosis to her boyfriend. At this time, the urgency of disclosing her diagnosis should depend on how comfortable she feels in discussing her illness with others and not on how acutely ill she becomes.

## 81 Correct answer—B

The nurse has a legal and ethical responsibility to keep G.'s diagnosis confidential. Yet she also must be sensitive to the needs of the family members who care about the patient. Asking family members, "What have you been told?" helps the nurse assess their understanding of the situation and puts her in a position to clarify information that the family members have but do not understand. Information that the patient does not wish to reveal should not be disclosed. Although the nurse cannot discuss the patient's diagnosis, refusing to address the mother's concerns will only heighten her anxiety. Telling the mother that her daughter is seriously ill borders on disclosure and is therefore inappropriate. Asking the mother "Do you have any thoughts about what your daugher's diagnosis might be?" serves no purpose because the nurse is legally and ethically constrained from confirming any thoughts about the diagnosis.

## 82  Correct answer—D

By acknowledging the patient's difficult decision, the nurse demonstrates empathy and acceptance and lets the patient know that she is sensitive to her feelings. Asking the patient to explore the positive results of revealing her illness may help the patient express her underlying feelings, such as her desire for parental support during this difficult time. Allowing the patient to verbalize the positive and negative aspects of telling her parents will provide her with a clear picture of the possible outcomes of her disclosure. The nurse should demonstrate care and sensitivity and not use clichés ("Everyone is going to die at some time") or judge the patient's behavior ("I don't think you are giving your parents a fair chance" or "How do you feel about keeping something so important from them?").

## 83  Correct answer—C

Because a history of violent behavior is a predictor of future violence, the nurse should review the patient's previous history and note any violent episodes. She should check carefully for precipitating factors leading to violence, such as altercations with strangers, and characteristic indicators of impending violence, such as combative gestures. Such information will help staff members plan safe, effective interventions to prevent and control the patient's violent behavior. Although other aspects of the patient's history, such as previous diagnoses, length of hospitalizations, and hallucinations are helpful in understanding the patient's overall needs, ensuring the patient's and others' safety is a priority.

## 84  Correct answer—D

An agitated, potentially violent patient should initially be given sufficient space to avoid making him feel closed in or threatened. The nurse should observe the patient from a safe distance and interact, when necessary, in a calm voice. Confrontation and restraint should be avoided if possible. If verbal attempts to reduce the patient's agitation are ineffective, the nurse can suggest that the patient go to his room for some quiet time. A patient should not be threatened with restraint or seclusion but told matter-of-factly that staff members will help him control his behavior if necessary. If the patient should become unexpectedly violent, the nurse should call on the help of other staff members to restrain the patient to protect him from himself and others.

## 85 Correct answer—A

In many instances, the nurse can diffuse impending violence by helping the patient identify and express his feelings of anger and anxiety. Such statements as "You seem pretty upset. How can I help?" and "What happened to get you this angry?" may help the patient verbalize his feelings rather than act upon them. Close interaction with the patient in a quiet activity may place the nurse at risk for injury should the patient become suddenly violent. An agitated and potentially violent patient should not be left alone or unsupervised because the danger of his acting out is too great. The patient should be placed in seclusion only after other interventions have been tried unsuccessfully or the patient himself requests it. Unlocked seclusion can be helpful for some patients because it reduces environmental stimuli and provides the patient with a feeling of security.

## 86 Correct answer—B

A well-coordinated plan of action is needed to restrain a patient while protecting both the patient and staff from injury. Restraint procedures should be clearly established and practiced as part of orientation and inservice training. The best plans include a designated leader and four or five (not seven or eight) staff members to restrain and medicate the patient. The leader should speak to the patient and calmly tell him why he is being restrained. A patient should be approached from the sides, not face-to-face, which is commonly viewed as a direct threat. Although the staff should act as quickly as possible to restrain the patient, doing so without a well-designed plan may be disastrous. After the patient is restrained, the nurse can administer a PRN medication, such as chlorpromazine, for agitation.

## 87 Correct answer—D

A show of force by several staff members approaching an agitated patient often is sufficient to control the patient's behavior. Avoiding restraints whenever possible is safer for both the patient and staff. If a patient agrees to go into seclusion on his own, he should be allowed to do so, but staff members should accompany him to the seclusion room to ensure safety. The amount of time spent in seclusion typically is determined by the patient's ability to control his behavior. Stepping back from the patient—whether to observe him or to allow him to go to the seclusion room—weakens the show of force and may exacerbate his behavior.

## 88 Correct answer—C

Releasing a patient from seclusion must be done carefully. The nurse should begin by opening the seclusion room door periodically to evaluate the patient's level of control. If the patient can follow instructions and remain in open seclusion as requested, she can allow him greater freedom. The nurse should tell the patient in clear terms that inability to follow restrictions will mean a return to seclusion. Allowing the patient to leave but remaining at a safe distance, or allowing the patient to leave after securing a verbal contract, is not the most effective or safest way to release a patient; the patient should be observed for some time before he is allowed to leave the seclusion area. To ensure safety, no one should enter the seclusion room until the patient is clearly under control.

## 89 Correct answer—B

Haloperidol is associated with a high incidence of extrapyramidal side effects. The nurse should assess the patient for evidence of dystonic reactions, parkinsonian symptoms, and akathisia. Early recognition is important because such side effects are reversible. Treatment may involve dosage reduction or the administration of an antiparkinsonian medication, such as amantadine (Symmetrel), benztropine (Cogentin), trihexyphenidyl (Artane), or procyclidine (Kemadrin). The incidence of sedation, cardiovascular effects, dizziness, orthostatic hypotension, and anticholinergic effects is low for haloperidol therapy.

## 90 Correct answer—D

A patient has a legal right to refuse treatment. The nurse should be familiar with the state laws and hospital policies regarding this issue. If, after encouragement, the patient continues to refuse the medication and his behavior presents no immediate threat to himself or others, the nurse should record the refusal and report it to appropriate staff members. The patient's behavior then should be closely monitored. The nurse also should attempt to determine why the patient is refusing the medication. Many times, a patient refuses to take medication because of the drug's side effects, such as dry mouth or drowsiness. If this is the case, the physician may alter the dosage or change the drug to promote compliance with the medication regimen. Administering a medication by injection against a patient's wishes is a violation of the patient's right to refuse treatment. If the patient refuses one type of medication, he probably will refuse an as-needed medication as well. Chastising the patient by saying his behavior is negative is a subtle attempt to coerce the patient and is therefore inappropriate.

## 91  Correct answer—C

A tolerant, attentive approach is essential when interacting with a confused older patient. Reassurance and repeated orientation to her new surroundings will help reduce the patient's anxiety, which is related to the change in environment and possibly compounded by age-related sensory deficits. Leaving D. alone, especially with dimmed lights, is inadvisable because this setting will increase, not decrease, her confusion. After the patient's anxiety has lessened and her perceptions clear, a call from her daughter may be beneficial. Introductions should be limited to her roommate, if applicable, and those working directly with the patient. D. will need time to adjust to her new surroundings and the staff members.

## 92  Correct answer—B

Therapeutic communication aims at acknowledging the patient's feelings and encouraging further ventilation of those feelings. In this situation, the nurse expresses empathy ("It must be frightening to hear your mother say she is going to die"), then makes herself available and encourages expression of feelings. Asking the daughter whether she can care for her mother at home will serve only to increase her guilt over the situation. Telling the daughter not to feel guilty does not encourage her to discuss how she feels. Although it is true that many patients in nursing homes are agitated and confused initially, stating this fact without allowing the daughter to express her concerns is nontherapeutic.

## 93  Correct answer—D

Because placing a relative in a nursing home can be difficult and stressful for the patient's family, the nurse should encourage the individual family members to protect their own health and well-being and support them in their decisions. Acknowledging the daughter's difficulty in deciding to place her mother in a home demonstrates empathy and validates her feelings. Encouraging the daughter to call and telling her that the nurse will keep in touch provides added reassurance that her mother will receive constant care and that it is okay to take care of herself. Acknowledging the daughter's difficulties without encouraging her to call or stating that the nurse will keep in touch does little to reassure the daughter that she has made the best decision. The nurse should not imply that the daughter's decision is wrong by questioning it.

## 94 Correct answer—A

A primary strategy when working with a confused older patient is to establish a predictable routine. Activities of daily living and other routine nursing care measures should occur at the same time each day as part of a structured, therapeutic milieu. This manipulation of the environment helps maintain reality orientation, reduces confusion, and promotes a sense of safety and security for the patient. Restraints should be avoided unless no other alternatives to protecting the patient from injury are available. Limiting the patient's decision-making opportunities would foster dependence, regression, and withdrawal and decrease her self-esteem. Reminiscing, which is commonly stimulated by a change in environment or anticipation of death, should not be discouraged because it is a significant part of aging.

## 95 Correct answer—A

Short-term memory loss is more common than long-term memory loss in older persons. This impairment, which may result from physiologic, psychological, and perceptual factors of aging, should be considered when planning the patient's care. For example, the nurse should anticipate the need for repeating instructions and other information to the patient and alert the staff and the patient's family to do likewise. Generally, a person's personality traits remain intact as he ages. Someone who has been negative and difficult to get along with throughout his life probably will remain so. The nurse should not assume that negativism is a shared trait among all elderly patients. Some of the negativity seen in these patients may be related to sensory deficits, short-term memory loss, and other anxiety-producing factors. Confusion does not automatically occur with aging; its occurrence in older patients indicates an underlying physical or psychiatric problem.

## 96 Correct answer—D

Tourette's syndrome is a chronic tic disorder characterized by compulsive behaviors, verbal outbursts, and muscular tics. Coprolalia, a phonic tic, is one of the manifestations of this disorder. A patient with coprolalia typically makes obscene and aggressive statements that are quite upsetting to those around him. Echolalia is the automatic repetition of another person's words. Echopraxia is the repetition of another's movement. Echolalia and echopraxia are sometimes seen in patients with schizophrenia. Dyslexia is inability to read, which often is related to organic brain syndrome or neurologic injury.

## 97 Correct answer—B

Haloperidol (Haldol) and other neuroleptic (antipsychotic) medications are used to control the tics and vocal utterances of patients with Tourette's syndrome. Diazepam (Valium), a muscle relaxant, and amantadine hydrochloride (Symmetrel), an antiparkisonian, anticholinergic, and antiviral agent, are not used in the treatment of Tourette's syndrome because neither drug affects the behavior associated with this condition. Phenelzine sulfate (Nardil), a monoamine oxidase inhibitor, is used primarily for patients who do not respond to tricyclic or other antidepressants.

## 98 Correct answer—D

The nurse should use this opportunity to acknowledge the nursing assistant's feelings and to foster group problem-solving skills. This situation is ideal for teaching the assistants about Tourette's syndrome and discussing strategies for handling the distress caused by the patient's obscene outbursts. Telling the assistant to treat everyone as equal, agreeing with her, or ignoring her comments does not promote learning or provide the assistant with new skills to better meet the patient's needs.

## 99 Correct answer—B

The most appropriate action in this situation is to sit silently beside the patient while he is crying, then ask him to describe his feelings once he is able to talk. By sitting beside him in this manner, the nurse shows that she accepts his need to grieve and that she is available for support. Asking the patient to describe his feelings demonstrates that she is willing to listen and validates the patient's feelings as well as the significance of the grieving process. Leaving the patient alone at this time is inappropriate because the nurse should attempt to help the patient to identify his feelings and to understand that crying about an anticipated loss is a normal part of grieving. Putting an arm around the patient is inadvisable unless the patient and the nurse both find touching comfortable and acceptable. Any form of distraction at this time is improper because it invalidates the patient's feelings.

## 100 Correct answer—A

The most therapeutic response is to reflect the patient's acknowledgment of the reality of his situation, then encourage him to explore his feelings about it. A Type I (insulin-dependent) diabetic, especially one who has undergone amputation, can never lead a normal life because of the constraints of his disease. Any discussion to the contrary is inappropriate. Saying "I can't believe how defeated you sound..." implies that the patient's feelings are unfounded and therefore invalid. Saying that the patient will soon be feeling like his old self again fails to explore the patient's feelings and may provide him with false reassurance about his expected recovery.

# Selected References

## Books

Arnold, E., and Boggs, K. *Interpersonal Relationships: Professional Communication Skills for Nurses.* Philadelphia: W.B. Saunders Co., 1989.

Beck, C., et al. *Mental Health–Psychiatric Nursing,* 2nd ed. St. Louis: C.V. Mosby Co., 1988.

Brenner, M. *Mental Health and Psychiatric Nursing.* Springhouse Notes series. Springhouse, Pa.: Springhouse Corp., 1988.

Burgess, A.W. *Psychiatric Nursing in the Hospital and the Community,* 5th ed. Englewood Cliffs, N.J.: Prentice-Hall, 1990.

Cook, J.S., and Fontaine, K.L. *Essentials of Mental Health Nursing.* Menlo Park, Calif.: Addison-Wesley, 1987.

DeVita, V.T., et al, eds. *AIDS: Etiology, Diagnosis, Treatment and Prevention,* 2nd ed. Philadelphia: J.B. Lippincott Co., 1988.

*Diagnostic and Statistical Manual of Mental Disorders (DSM-III-R),* 3rd edition—revised. Washington, D.C.: American Psychiatric Association, 1987.

Doenges, M.E., et al. *Psychiatric Care Plans: Guidelines for Client Care.* Philadelphia: F.A. Davis Co., 1988.

Estes, N.T., and Heinemann, M.E. *Alcoholism: Development, Consequences and Interventions,* 3rd ed. St. Louis: C.V. Mosby Co., 1986.

Govani, L.E., and Hayes, J.E. *Drugs and Nursing Implications,* 6th ed. Norwalk, Conn.: Appleton-Lange, 1988.

Haber, J., et al. *Comprehensive Psychiatric Nursing,* 3rd ed. New York: McGraw-Hill Book Co., 1987.

Hoff, L.A. *People in Crises: Understanding and Helping,* 3rd ed. Menlo Park, Calif.: Addison-Wesley, 1989.

Janosik, E.H., ed. *Crises Counseling: A Contemporary Approach.* Monterey, Calif.: Wadsworth, 1986.

Janosik, E., and Davies, L. *Psychiatric Mental Health Nursing,* 2nd ed. Boston: Jones & Bartlett, 1989.

Johnson, B.S. *Psychiatric–Mental Health Nursing: Adaptation and Growth.* Philadelphia: J.B. Lippincott Co., 1986.

Johnson, J.H., et al. *Approaches to Child Treatment.* New York: Pergamon, 1986.

Kaplan, H., and Sadock, B., eds. *Comprehensive Textbook of Psychiatry IV,* 5th ed, Vol. 1. Baltimore: Williams & Wilkens Co., 1989.

Kermes, M.D. *Mental Health in Late Life.* Boston: Jones & Bartlett Pub., 1986.

Malseed, R., and Harrigan, G. *Textbook of Pharmacology and Nursing Care.* Philadelphia: J.B. Lippincott Co., 1989.

McFarland, G., and Wasli, E. *Nursing Diagnoses and Process in Psychiatric–Mental Health Nursing.* Philadelphia: J.B. Lippincott Co., 1986.

Murray, R.B., and Huelskoetter, M.M. *Psychiatric/Mental Health Nursing—Giving Emotional Care,* 2nd ed. Norwalk, Conn.: Appleton & Lange, 1991.

Pasquali, E.A. et al. *Mental Health Nursing: A Holistic Approach,* 3rd ed. St. Louis: C.V. Mosby Co., 1989.

Perko, J., and Kreigh, H.Z. *Psychiatric and Mental Health Nursing,* 3rd ed. Norwalk, Conn.: Appleton & Lange, 1988.

Reighley, J.W. *Nursing Care Planning Guides for Mental Health.* Baltimore: Williams & Wilkens Co., 1988.

Roberts, M.C. *Pediatric Psychology-Psychological Interventions and Strategies for Pediatric Problems.* New York: Pergamon, 1986.

Schultz, J., and Dark, S. *Manual of Psychiatric Nursing Care Plans,* 3rd ed. Boston: Little, Brown & Co., 1990.

Shives, L.R. *Basic Concepts of Psychiatric–Mental Health Nursing.* Philadelphia: J.B. Lippincott Co., 1986.

*Springhouse Drug Reference.* Springhouse, Pa.: Springhouse Corp., 1988.

Stuart, G., and Sundeen, S. *Principles and Practice of Psychiatric Nursing,* 4th ed. St. Louis: Mosby-Year Book, Inc., 1991.

Wilson, H.S., and Kneisl, C.R. *Psychiatric Nursing,* 3rd ed. Menlo Park, Calif.: Addison-Wesley, 1988.

**Periodicals**

Laufman, J. "AIDS, Ethics, and the Truth," *American Journal of Nursing* 89(7):924-30, July 1989.

Williams, L. "Alzheimer's: The Need for Caring," *Journal of Gerontological Nursing* 12(2):20-28, February 1986.

# Index